I0839709

DIET

AND

DIABETES

THE ULTIMATE GUIDE TO A HEALTHY DIET FOR A DIABETIC PATIENT

DR. STIEN

© 2024 by Dr. Stien. All rights reserved.

No part of this book may be reproduced or utilized in any form or by any means, electronic or mechanical, including photocopying, recording, or by any information storage and retrieval system, without permission in writing from the publisher.

First Edition 2024

Published by Dr. Stien

CONTENTS

INTRODUCTION

Navigating the world of food and nutrition can be especially challenging when managing a condition like diabetes. With so much information out there, it can be hard to know what's truly helpful. This book is here to be your reliable guide.

In these pages, we'll explore the complex relationship between diet and diabetes, breaking down the science in an easy-to-understand and practical way. We'll look at different types of foods and how they affect blood glucose levels, helping you grasp the importance of portion sizes, meal planning, and maintaining a balanced diet.

We'll also clear up common myths about diabetes and diet, giving you evidence-based advice. You'll learn about the roles of carbohydrates, fats, proteins, and even the often overlooked micronutrients in managing diabetes effectively.

But this book is more than just a list of 'do's and 'don'ts'. It's about empowering you with the knowledge and tools you need to make informed decisions about your diet and health. It's about understanding that while diabetes is part of your life, it doesn't define you or limit you.

Whether you're newly diagnosed or have been managing diabetes for years, this book offers practical tips to help you live a healthy, fulfilling life. It's also a valuable resource for caregivers and healthcare professionals, providing a comprehensive overview of diet management in diabetes.

"Diet and Diabetes: The Ultimate Guide to a Healthy Diet for a Diabetic Patient" is not just a book; it's a call to action, a guide, and a resource. It stands as proof that with the right knowledge and tools, you can manage diabetes successfully. So, let's dive in and start this enlightening journey together.

Chapter 1: Understanding Diabetes

Introduction to Diabetes

Diabetes is a metabolic disorder that affects millions worldwide, marked by high blood sugar levels over a long period. It happens when the body either can't produce insulin or can't use it effectively. There are two main types: type 1 diabetes, where the body fails to produce insulin, and type 2 diabetes, where the body can't use insulin properly.

Poorly managed diabetes can lead to serious health issues like heart disease, stroke, kidney problems, eye issues, and nerve damage. That's why it's crucial to manage this chronic condition effectively to prevent these long-term complications.

Diet is a key player in managing diabetes. What you eat, when you eat, and how much you eat can greatly impact your blood sugar levels. Understanding the relationship between food and blood sugar is vital for anyone with diabetes. A balanced diet helps maintain healthy blood glucose levels, reduces the risk of complications, and improves overall well-being.

Carbohydrates have the most significant effect on blood sugar levels. When you eat carbs, they break down into glucose and enter your bloodstream. Managing carb intake is essential in diabetes management. But it's not just about cutting down on carbs; it's also about choosing the right kinds. Foods with a low glycemic index cause a slower, more gradual rise in blood sugar, making them better choices.

Protein and fats have little to no direct impact on blood sugar levels, but they should still be eaten in moderation. Too much fat, especially saturated and trans fats, can lead to weight gain and an increased risk of heart disease, which is especially concerning for those with diabetes.

Alongside diet, regular physical activity helps manage diabetes by boosting insulin sensitivity and lowering blood sugar levels. Maintaining a healthy weight also significantly reduces the risk of developing type 2 diabetes and helps manage the condition if you already have it.

Understanding how diet affects diabetes is a crucial step toward living healthily with this condition. It's about making informed food choices, balancing nutritious meals with physical activity, and making necessary lifestyle changes. With the right approach, diabetes can be effectively managed, allowing you to live a healthy and fulfilling life.

Types of Diabetes

The three primary types of diabetes are type 1 diabetes, type 2 diabetes and gestational diabetes.

Type 1 diabetes:
The exact cause of type 1 diabetes is not fully understood, but it is believed to be a combination of genetic predisposition and environmental factors.
Symptoms of type 1 diabetes often develop quickly and include excessive thirst, frequent urination, unexplained weight loss, fatigue, and blurred vision.

Type 2 Diabetes:

Type 2 diabetes is the most common form of diabetes and is characterized by insulin resistance, where the body's cells do not respond effectively to insulin. This leads to high blood sugar levels.

Type 2 diabetes is often linked to lifestyle factors such as poor diet, lack of physical activity, and obesity. Genetics and family history also play a role in its development.

Symptoms of type 2 diabetes may develop gradually and include increased thirst, frequent urination, fatigue, blurred vision, and slow wound healing.

Gestational Diabetes:

Gestational diabetes occurs during pregnancy and is characterized by high blood sugar levels that develop for the first time during pregnancy.

Gestational diabetes is believed to be caused by hormonal changes during pregnancy that affect insulin function.

Many women with gestational diabetes may not experience any noticeable symptoms. However, some may experience increased thirst, frequent urination, and fatigue.

Other Types of diabetes:

Other less common types of diabetes include monogenic diabetes, which is caused by a mutation in a single gene, and secondary diabetes, which is a result of another medical condition or medication.

The causes and treatments for these types of diabetes vary depending on the specific condition and underlying factors.

Understanding the different types of diabetes is essential for individuals living with the condition, as it guides personalized treatment plans and lifestyle adjustments. Proper management of diabetes, including dietary choices, plays a crucial role in maintaining blood sugar levels within a healthy range and reducing the risk

Complications and Management

Living with diabetes requires careful management to prevent or delay the onset of various complications that can arise from uncontrolled blood sugar levels. Understanding these complications and how to effectively manage them is crucial for individuals with diabetes to lead a healthy and fulfilling life.

Types of Diabetes Complications

Acute Complications:

Acute complications of diabetes can occur suddenly and require immediate attention. The two main acute complications are:

Hypoglycemia:

Hypoglycemia, or low blood sugar, can result from excessive insulin or oral diabetes medication, insufficient food intake, or excessive physical activity.

Symptoms include shakiness, sweating, confusion, and in severe cases, loss of consciousness.

Management involves consuming fast-acting carbohydrates like glucose tablets, fruit juice, or candy to raise blood sugar levels quickly.

<u>Hyperglycemia:</u>

Hyperglycemia, or high blood sugar, can be caused by factors such as missed insulin doses, overeating, illness, or stress.

Symptoms may include increased thirst, frequent urination, fatigue, and blurred vision.

Treatment involves adjusting insulin doses, monitoring blood sugar levels closely, and staying hydrated.

<u>Chronic Complications:</u>

Chronic complications of diabetes develop gradually over time and can affect various organs and systems in the body. The key chronic complications include:

<u>Cardiovascular Complications:</u>

Diabetes significantly increases the risk of heart disease, stroke, and peripheral vascular disease.

Management involves maintaining healthy blood pressure and cholesterol levels, regular exercise, a balanced diet, and avoiding smoking.

<u>Neuropathy</u>

Diabetic neuropathy is nerve damage that can lead to pain, numbness, tingling, or weakness in the hands and feet.

Management includes blood sugar control, pain management strategies, and regular foot care.

Nephropathy

Diabetic nephropathy is kidney damage that can progress to kidney failure.

Management includes blood pressure control, monitoring kidney function, and following a kidney-friendly diet.

Retinopathy

Diabetic retinopathy is a leading cause of blindness in adults and is characterized by damage to the blood vessels in the retina.

Management involves regular eye exams, blood sugar control, blood pressure management, and laser treatment in some cases.

Foot Complications

Diabetic foot problems can result from nerve damage, poor circulation, and decreased immune function.

Management includes daily foot inspections, proper foot care, wearing appropriate footwear, and seeking prompt treatment for any foot issues.

Management Strategies

Blood Sugar Control:

Consistent blood sugar monitoring and maintaining target levels are essential to prevent complications.

This includes regular self-monitoring, medication adherence, and adjustments to diet and exercise as needed.

Nutritional Management:

A healthy diet plays a crucial role in diabetes management and can help control blood sugar levels.

Focus on a balanced diet rich in whole grains, fruits, vegetables, lean proteins, and healthy fats while limiting sugar and processed foods.

Physical Activity:

Regular exercise can improve blood sugar control, reduce cardiovascular risk, and enhance overall well-being.

Aim for a combination of aerobic exercise, strength training, and physical exercise.

Chapter 2: The Diabetic Diet

Principles of a Healthy Diabetic Diet

Below are some basic principles every diabetic patient should adhere to in order to improve their quality of life.

Balance carbohydrates:

Carbohydrates have the biggest impact on blood sugar levels, so it is important for individuals with diabetes to monitor their carbohydrate intake. Focus on choosing complex carbohydrates such as whole grains, fruits, and vegetables, and limit simple sugars and highly processed foods.

Include protein:

Protein helps to stabilize blood sugar levels and keeps you feeling full. Include sources of lean protein such as poultry, fish, tofu, beans, and low-fat dairy in your meals.

Choose healthy fats:

Fats are an important part of a balanced diet, but it is important to choose healthy fats such as olive oil, avocado, nuts, and seeds. Limit saturated and trans fats found in processed foods and fatty meats.

Eat plenty of fiber:

Fiber can help control blood sugar levels and improve digestion. Include plenty of fiber-rich foods such as whole grains, fruits, vegetables, and legumes in your meals.

Watch portion sizes:

Monitoring portion sizes is important for managing blood sugar levels and maintaining a healthy weight. Use measuring cups and spoons to control portion sizes and practice mindful eating to avoid overeating.

Be mindful of timing:

Spread out your meals and snacks throughout the day to keep your blood sugar levels stable. It is also important to monitor your blood sugar levels before and after meals to understand how certain foods affect your body.

Stay hydrated:

Drink plenty of water throughout the day to stay hydrated and support healthy blood sugar levels. Limit sugary drinks and opt for water, herbal tea, or unsweetened beverages instead.

Work with a registered dietitian:

A registered dietitian can help you create a personalized meal plan and provide guidance on managing your diabetes through healthy eating. They can also help you navigate dining out, grocery shopping, and making healthy food choices.

By following these principles of a healthy diabetic diet, individuals with diabetes can better manage their blood sugar levels, improve their overall health, and reduce the risk of complications associated with the condition. Incorporating a balanced diet, regular exercise, and working closely with healthcare providers can help individuals with diabetes live healthy and fulfilling lives.

Carbohydrate Counting

Carbohydrate counting is a method used by individuals with diabetes to manage their blood sugar levels by tracking the amount of carbohydrates they consume. This technique is particularly helpful for individuals who require insulin or other medications that are dependent on carbohydrate intake. In this section, we will provide a comprehensive overview of carbohydrate counting, including its benefits, how to get started, and practical tips for incorporating this approach into your daily routine.

What is Carbohydrate Counting?

Carbohydrate counting involves keeping track of the number of carbohydrates in the foods you eat and matching them to the amount of insulin or medication you need. Carbohydrates are the macronutrient that has the most significant impact on blood sugar levels, so by monitoring and controlling carbohydrate intake, individuals with diabetes can better manage their blood sugar levels.

Benefits of Carbohydrate Counting

<u>Improved blood sugar control:</u>
By accurately tracking carbohydrate intake and matching it with insulin or medication doses, individuals with diabetes can better manage their blood sugar levels and reduce the risk of fluctuations.

<u>Flexibility in diet:</u>
Carbohydrate counting allows individuals to have more flexibility in their food choices while still maintaining good blood sugar control. It is a more personalized approach to meal planning that takes into account individual preferences and needs.

<u>Increased awareness of food choices:</u> Carbohydrate counting encourages individuals to be more mindful of the types and amounts of carbohydrates they consume, leading to healthier food choices and better overall health.

Getting Started with Carbohydrate Counting

<u>Understand carb counting basics:</u>

Learn about the different types of carbohydrates (simple vs. complex), how they affect blood sugar levels, and how to accurately measure portion sizes.

<u>Consult with a registered dietitian:</u>

A registered dietitian can help you create a personalized meal plan, set carbohydrate goals, and provide guidance on how to count carbohydrates effectively.

<u>Use carbohydrate counting tools:</u>

Utilize resources such as food labels, carbohydrate counting apps, and books with carbohydrate counts for common foods to help you track your carbohydrate intake accurately.

<u>Monitor blood sugar levels:</u>

Regularly check your blood sugar levels before and after meals to see how different amounts of carbohydrates impact your readings. Adjust your carbohydrate intake and insulin doses accordingly.

Practical Tips for Carbohydrate Counting

<u>Measure portion sizes:</u>

Use measuring cups, a food scale, or visual aids to accurately measure portion sizes and track your carbohydrate intake.

<u>Keep a food diary:</u>

Write down the foods you eat, along with their carbohydrate content, to help you monitor your intake and identify patterns in your blood sugar levels.

<u>Plan meals and snacks in advance:</u>

Plan your meals and snacks ahead of time to ensure you meet your carbohydrate goals and have a balanced diet throughout the day.

<u>Be consistent:</u>

Try to eat a consistent amount of carbohydrates at each meal and snack to help maintain stable blood sugar levels.

By incorporating carbohydrate counting into your daily routine, individuals with diabetes can gain better control over their blood sugar levels, improve their overall health, and reduce the risk of complications associated with the condition. This personalized approach to meal planning provides individuals with the tools and knowledge they need to make informed food choices and manage their diabetes effectively.

Protein and Fat in Diabetic Diet

Proteins and fat also play a crucial role in managing diabetes effectively. A well-balanced diet that is rich in both can help stabilize blood sugar levels and prevent complications associated with diabetes. Let us explore the importance of protein and fat in a diabetic diet, as well as provide practical tips for incorporating these nutrients into your daily meals.

Protein in a Diabetic Diet

Protein is essential for maintaining and repairing body tissues, supporting immune function, and providing a feeling of fullness after meals. Including adequate amounts of protein in a diabetic diet can help regulate blood sugar levels and prevent spikes in glucose.

Sources of Protein:

Good sources of protein include lean meats such as poultry, fish, and tofu, as well as dairy products like Greek yogurt and cottage cheese. Plant-based sources of protein, such as beans, lentils, and quinoa, are also excellent options for individuals with diabetes.

Recommendations:

It is recommended that individuals with diabetes consume a moderate amount of protein at each meal, as excessive protein intake can lead to increased blood sugar levels. Aim to include lean sources of protein in your diet and avoid processed meats high in saturated fat and sodium.

Fat in a Diabetic Diet

Healthy fats are an essential component of a balanced diet for individuals with diabetes. Healthy fats support brain function, hormone production, and nutrient absorption, while also providing a source of long-lasting energy.

Types of Fats:

There are three main types of fats: unsaturated fats, saturated fats, and trans fats. Unsaturated fats, found in foods like avocados, nuts, and olive oil, are heart-healthy fats that can help lower cholesterol levels and reduce inflammation. Saturated fats, found in foods like butter, red meat, and cheese, should be consumed in moderation to prevent negative health effects. Trans fats, found in processed foods like fried foods and packaged snacks, should be avoided entirely.

Recommendations:

Incorporate sources of healthy fats into your meals, such as fatty fish like salmon, flaxseeds, and nuts. Limit your intake of saturated and trans fats, as they can increase the risk of heart disease and worsen diabetes symptoms. Focus on consuming whole, nutrient-dense foods that are rich in healthy fats to support overall health and well-being.

Conclusion:

By incorporating lean sources of protein and healthy fats into your meals, you can stabilize blood sugar levels, improve insulin sensitivity, and reduce the risk of complications associated with diabetes. Remember to focus on whole, nutritious foods that support your overall health and well-being, and also don't forget to consult with a healthcare provider or registered dietitian for personalized nutrition recommendations.

Fruits and Vegetables for Diabetics

Incorporating a variety of fruits and vegetables into a diabetic diet is essential for managing blood sugar levels, maintaining overall health, and reducing the risk of complications associated with diabetes. In this section, we shall delve into the benefits of consuming fruits and vegetables for individuals with diabetes, as well as provide recommendations on how to include these nutrient-rich foods in your daily meals.

Benefits of Fruits and Vegetables for Diabetics

Fruits and vegetables are low in calories and high in essential nutrients, such as fiber, vitamins, and minerals. These foods are also rich in antioxidants, which help protect the body from oxidative stress and inflammation. Consuming a wide range of fruits and vegetables can aid in weight management, improve blood sugar control, and reduce the risk of developing chronic diseases, such as heart disease and stroke.

Impact on Blood Sugar Levels

Certain fruits, such as berries, apples, and citrus fruits, have a lower glycemic index, meaning they cause a gradual rise in blood sugar levels compared to high-sugar fruits like watermelon and pineapple. Vegetables like leafy greens, broccoli, and bell peppers are also low in carbohydrates and have minimal impact on blood sugar levels. Including a mix of both low-glycemic fruits and non-starchy vegetables in your diet can help regulate blood sugar levels and prevent spikes in glucose.

Recommendations for Fruits and Vegetables

Focus on Variety:

Aim to consume a diverse range of fruits and vegetables to ensure you are getting a wide array of nutrients.

Portion Control:

Be mindful of portion sizes when consuming fruits, especially those higher in sugar. Stick to small servings to avoid blood sugar spikes.

Incorporate Fiber:

Fruits and vegetables are excellent sources of dietary fiber, which can help regulate blood sugar levels, improve digestion, and promote satiety.

Choose Whole Foods:

Opt for whole fruits and vegetables over processed or canned options, as they tend to have added sugars, sodium, and preservatives.

Experiment with Cooking Methods:

Try different cooking methods, such as roasting, steaming, or grilling, to add variety and enhance the flavor of your fruits and vegetables.

Conclusion:

Fruits and vegetables are essential components of a healthy diabetic diet, providing a wide range of nutrients and health benefits. By incorporating a variety of colorful fruits and vegetables into your meals, you can support overall health, improve blood sugar control, and reduce the risk of complications associated with diabetes. Remember to prioritize whole, nutrient-dense foods and consult with a healthcare provider or registered dietitian for personalized nutrition recommendations. Embrace the power of fruits and vegetables in managing your diabetes and enjoy the delicious flavors and nourishment they provide.

Chapter 3: Meal Planning for Diabetics

Meal Timing and Portion Control

In the management of diabetes, dietary choices play a crucial role in regulating blood sugar levels. Two key factors that significantly impact diabetes control are meal timing and portion control. Understanding how these factors influence blood glucose levels can empower individuals to make informed choices for better health outcomes.

Meal Timing

Proper meal timing is essential for individuals with diabetes to maintain stable blood sugar levels throughout the day. Consistency in meal timing helps regulate insulin levels and prevents blood sugar spikes and crashes. Here are some key points regarding meal timing:

Regular Meals:

Eating meals at consistent times each day helps the body anticipate and manage glucose levels effectively.

Balanced Meal Spacing:

Spreading meals evenly throughout the day can help control blood sugar levels and prevent extreme fluctuations.

<u>Pre-Meal Planning:</u>

Planning meals in advance allows for better control over carbohydrate intake and promotes healthier food choices.

<u>Post-Meal Monitoring:</u>

Monitoring blood sugar levels after meals can provide valuable insights into how different foods affect glucose levels and help adjust dietary choices accordingly.

Portion Control

Controlling portion sizes is vital for managing diabetes as it directly impacts blood sugar levels and weight management. Proper portion control can help individuals with diabetes maintain a healthy weight and improve overall well-being. Here are some strategies for portion control:

<u>Plate Method:</u>

Using the plate method, individuals can visually divide their plates to include appropriate proportions of carbohydrates, proteins, and vegetables for balanced meals.

<u>Measuring Tools:</u>

Using measuring cups, spoons, and food scales can help accurately portion out foods and track caloric intake.

<u>Mindful Eating:</u>

Practicing mindful eating techniques, such as eating slowly and savoring each bite, can help prevent overeating and promote better portion control.

<u>Reading Labels:</u>

Understanding portion sizes on food labels and nutritional information can assist in making informed choices about portion control and overall dietary intake.

<u>Conclusion:</u>

Incorporating mindful meal timing and practicing portion control are essential components of a comprehensive diabetes management plan. By understanding the impact of meal timing and portion control on blood sugar levels, individuals can make conscious dietary choices to better manage their diabetes and improve their overall quality of life.

Creating a Balanced Plate

A balanced plate is a healthy meal that includes a variety of foods in appropriate portions. It's a simple way to ensure you are getting the nutrients your body needs.

For individuals with diabetes, managing their diet is a critical aspect of maintaining good health and managing blood sugar levels effectively. Crafting a balanced plate is a fundamental principle in diabetes management, as it helps regulate blood glucose levels, promotes overall well-being, and reduces the risk of diabetes-related complications. This chapter will delve into the essential components of a balanced plate tailored for individuals with diabetes, providing insights and guidelines to make informed dietary choices for optimal health outcomes.

Components of a Balanced Plate for Diabetics

<u>Carbohydrates:</u>

As stated earlier, carbohydrates have a direct impact on blood sugar levels, making carb management crucial for individuals with diabetes. Opt for complex carbohydrates with a low glycemic index to prevent rapid spikes in blood sugar. Examples include whole grains, legumes, fruits, and vegetables. Portion control is essential, as even healthy carbohydrates can affect blood glucose levels when consumed in large quantities.

<u>Proteins:</u>

Proteins are essential for maintaining muscle mass, promoting satiety, and regulating blood sugar levels. Lean protein sources such as skinless poultry, fish, tofu, legumes, and low-fat dairy products are ideal choices for individuals with diabetes. Including protein in each meal can help stabilize blood sugar levels and prevent sharp fluctuations.

<u>Healthy Fats:</u>

Incorporating healthy fats into your diet is beneficial for heart health and overall well-being. Opt for sources of unsaturated fats such as nuts, seeds, avocados, olive oil, and fatty fish like salmon. While fats are calorie-dense, consuming them in moderation can help improve insulin sensitivity and support cardiovascular health.

<u>Fiber:</u>

Dietary fiber plays a crucial role in regulating blood sugar levels, promoting digestive health, and enhancing satiety. Aim to include ample fiber in your meals through foods like fruits, vegetables, whole grains, legumes, and nuts. Fiber can slow down the absorption of glucose, preventing rapid spikes in blood sugar levels.

Snacking Smart

One aspect that can significantly impact blood sugar control is the choice and timing of snacks. We will now explore how individuals with diabetes can make smart snacking choices to help manage their condition effectively.

Understanding Snacking for Diabetics

<u>Role of Snacks:</u>

Snacks play a vital role in managing diabetes by preventing extreme blood sugar fluctuations between meals.

<u>Importance of Smart Snacking</u>:

Choosing the right snacks can help individuals maintain steady energy levels, control hunger, and prevent overeating during main meals.

Characteristics of Diabetic-Friendly Snacks

<u>Low Glycemic Index (GI)</u>: Opt for snacks with a low GI to prevent rapid spikes in blood sugar levels.

<u>Balanced Macronutrients</u>: Include a combination of carbohydrates, protein, and healthy fats to promote satiety and maintain stable blood sugar levels.

<u>Portion Control</u>: Pay attention to portion sizes to avoid excessive calorie intake, which can affect blood sugar control.

Smart Snack Ideas for Diabetics

<u>Fresh Fruits and Vegetables</u>:

Opt for whole fruits and vegetables, as they are rich in fiber and essential nutrients.

<u>Nuts and Seeds</u>:

Almonds, walnuts, chia seeds, and flaxseeds are excellent choices due to their healthy fats, protein, and fiber content.

<u>Greek Yogurt</u>:

High in protein and low in sugar, Greek yogurt can be a satisfying and nutritious snack.

<u>Whole Grain Crackers with Hummus:</u>

This combination provides a balance of carbohydrates, protein, and healthy fats.

Strategies for Successful Snacking

<u>Be Mindful:</u> Pay attention to hunger cues and avoid emotional eating.

<u>Plan Ahead:</u> Keep diabetic-friendly snacks readily available to prevent impulsive, unhealthy choices.

<u>Read Labels:</u> Check nutritional information for sugar content and portion sizes.

Timing and Frequency of Snacks

<u>Mid-Morning and Afternoon Snacks:</u> Consuming snacks between meals can help maintain energy levels and prevent blood sugar drops.

<u>Pre-Bedtime Snack:</u> A light snack before bed can prevent nighttime hypoglycemia.

<u>Conclusion</u>

Smart snacking plays a vital role in managing diabetes so it should be done properly as overindulgence will ultimately lead to a worse outcome.

Chapter 4: Understanding Food Labels

Decoding Nutritional Facts

Every meal choice carries profound implications for blood sugar regulation, making it imperative to unravel the complexities encoded within food labels. This section embarks on a comprehensive exploration of nutritional facts, equipping diabetics with the knowledge and insight needed to navigate dietary decisions with precision and confidence.

Understanding Serving Sizes

At the heart of interpreting nutritional facts lies a nuanced understanding of serving sizes. Often underestimated or misunderstood, serving sizes wield significant influence over caloric and nutrient intake. Misjudging serving sizes can lead to inadvertent overconsumption, disrupting blood sugar levels and thwarting diabetes management efforts. By mastering the art of accurately discerning serving sizes, individuals empower themselves to make informed dietary choices that promote optimal health and well-being.

Interpreting Macronutrients

Macronutrients—carbohydrates, proteins, and fats—form the foundation of dietary composition and exert profound effects on blood glucose regulation and as you know carbohydrates, in particular, demand meticulous attention due to their primary role in determining postprandial glycemic responses. Yet, the intricate interplay between macronutrients necessitates a holistic approach to dietary assessment. Proteins and fats, though less directly impactful on blood sugar, wield considerable influence over satiety, metabolic health, and overall nutritional balance. By embracing a nuanced understanding of macronutrients, individuals can tailor their dietary choices to optimize blood sugar control and enhance overall health outcomes.

Decoding Carbohydrates

Carbohydrates stand as the linchpin of diabetes management, demanding meticulous scrutiny and strategic planning. Within the realm of carbohydrates, discerning total carbohydrate content, dietary fiber, and sugars unveils essential insights into food composition and metabolic impact. While total carbohydrates provide a comprehensive view of available energy sources, dietary fiber emerges as a crucial ally in mitigating postprandial glycemic excursions and fostering metabolic stability. Furthermore, distinguishing between naturally occurring sugars and added sugars empowers individuals to make discerning choices that prioritize nutrient density and minimize glycemically disruptive ingredients.

Navigating Fats

Fats, often vilified in the context of chronic disease management, merit nuanced consideration in the landscape of diabetes care. Beyond their caloric density, the quality and composition of dietary fats exert profound effects on metabolic health and cardiovascular risk. Unsaturated fats, celebrated for their cardioprotective properties, offer a spectrum of health benefits, from reducing inflammation to improving lipid profiles. Conversely, saturated and trans fats pose significant health risks, exacerbating insulin resistance and promoting a pro-inflammatory milieu. By embracing a paradigm that prioritizes the consumption of healthful fats while minimizing intake of deleterious varieties, individuals can cultivate dietary patterns that support optimal metabolic function and mitigate long-term complications associated with diabetes.

Evaluating Sodium and Hidden Culprits

Sodium, though often overshadowed by discussions of macronutrients, emerges as a critical determinant of cardiovascular health and overall well-being in individuals with diabetes. Excessive sodium intake exacerbates hypertension, amplifies cardiovascular risk, and undermines metabolic stability. Furthermore, hidden culprits such as artificial sweeteners, preservatives, and flavor enhancers may permeate processed foods, posing insidious threats to blood sugar control and metabolic health. By adopting a vigilant stance towards sodium intake and cultivating a discerning eye for hidden ingredients, individuals can safeguard against dietary pitfalls and forge a path towards sustained health and vitality.

Conclusion:

Deciphering nutritional facts transcends mere label reading; it embodies a journey of empowerment, enlightenment, and self-discovery. By mastering the intricacies of serving sizes, macronutrients, and hidden ingredients, individuals with diabetes embark on a transformative odyssey towards optimal health and well-being. Armed with knowledge, awareness, and the tools of discernment, they navigate the dietary landscape with confidence, resilience, and unwavering determination. In this pursuit, they transcend the confines of illness to embrace a life rich in vitality, vitality, and boundless possibility.

Understanding Ingredients

Every ingredient holds the potential to influence blood sugar regulation, metabolic health, and overall well-being. We will now embark on a comprehensive exploration of ingredients, illuminating the biochemical intricacies that underpin their impact on diabetes management. Through a nuanced understanding of ingredients, individuals with diabetes can navigate the culinary landscape with confidence, fostering a symbiotic relationship between nourishment and wellness.

Dissecting Carbohydrates

By discerning the glycemic index and glycemic load of carbohydrate-containing ingredients, individuals can tailor their dietary choices to optimize metabolic outcomes while prioritizing nutrient density and satiety.

Embracing Fiber

Fiber, often heralded as the unsung hero of diabetes-friendly nutrition, warrants meticulous attention in ingredient selection. Beyond its role in promoting gastrointestinal health and satiety, dietary fiber exerts significant metabolic benefits, including attenuating postprandial glycemic excursions and modulating insulin sensitivity. By incorporating fiber-rich ingredients such as whole grains, legumes, fruits, and vegetables into their culinary repertoire, individuals can cultivate dietary patterns that foster metabolic stability and long-term health.

Navigating Sugars

Sugars, both natural and added, occupy a contentious space in the dietary landscape of diabetes management. While naturally occurring sugars in whole foods are accompanied by fiber, vitamins, and minerals, added sugars permeate processed foods with little nutritional value and potent glycemic impact. By scrutinizing ingredient lists for sources of added sugars—such as high-fructose corn syrup, cane sugar, and various syrups—individuals can mitigate the risk of blood sugar spikes and cultivate a dietary environment conducive to metabolic health.

Unveiling Fats

Fats, often shrouded in misconception and ambiguity, wield considerable influence over metabolic health and cardiovascular risk in individuals with diabetes. Distinguishing between healthful fats—such as monounsaturated and polyunsaturated fats—and deleterious varieties— such as saturated and trans fats—forms the cornerstone of informed ingredient selection. By incorporating sources of healthful fats, such as avocados, nuts, seeds, and fatty fish, into their culinary repertoire, individuals can optimize lipid profiles, attenuate inflammation, and mitigate cardiovascular risk factors associated with diabetes.

Exploring Protein Sources

Proteins, the building blocks of cellular function and repair, play a multifaceted role in diabetes management. Beyond their satiating properties and potential impact on postprandial glycemia, proteins influence metabolic health through modulation of insulin sensitivity and secretion. By prioritizing lean sources of protein—such as poultry, fish, tofu, legumes, and low-fat dairy—individuals can optimize their dietary composition, support muscle health, and promote metabolic resilience in the face of diabetes-related challenges.

<u>Conclusion:</u>

Understanding ingredients transcends mere label reading; it embodies a journey of enlightenment, empowerment, and culinary creativity. By dissecting the biochemical intricacies of carbohydrates, fiber, sugars, fats, and proteins, individuals with diabetes embark on a transformative odyssey towards optimal health and well-being. Armed with knowledge, awareness, and the tools of discernment, they navigate the culinary landscape with confidence, resilience, and unwavering determination. In this pursuit, they transcend the confines of illness to embrace a life rich in nourishment, vitality, and boundless possibility.

Identifying Hidden Sugars

While some sugars are easily recognizable, many hide in processed foods under different names. Unveiling these hidden sugars empowers individuals to make informed dietary choices, promoting better blood sugar control and overall health.

The Hidden Sugar Epidemic

Sugar is ubiquitous in the modern diet, lurking in foods ranging from breakfast cereals to salad dressings. However, not all sources of sugar are obvious. Manufacturers often use various names for sugar to disguise its presence, such as sucrose, fructose, glucose, and high-fructose corn syrup (HFCS). Additionally, ingredients like maltodextrin, dextrose, and fruit juice concentrates are covert sources of sugar.

Identifying Hidden Sugars

Read Labels: Learning to decipher food labels is essential. Look beyond the "sugar" line and scan the ingredients list for any aliases of sugar. The higher up a sugar source is listed, the more of it the product contains.

<u>Watch for -ose Endings:</u>

Ingredients ending in "-ose" typically indicate sugars, such as fructose, glucose, and sucrose.

<u>Beware of Syrups and Concentrates:</u>

Ingredients like corn syrup, malt syrup, rice syrup, and fruit juice concentrate are concentrated sources of sugar.

<u>Carb Count:</u>

Carbohydrates break down into sugars during digestion. Even foods labeled as "low sugar" may contain high levels of carbohydrates, which can affect blood sugar levels.

<u>Assess Serving Sizes:</u>

Manufacturers often manipulate serving sizes to make products appear lower in sugar. Be mindful of portion sizes and how they impact sugar intake.

Impact on Blood Sugar Control

Hidden sugars can lead to spikes in blood sugar levels, complicating diabetes management. By identifying and reducing hidden sugar intake, individuals can stabilize their blood sugar levels, reducing the risk of diabetic complications and promoting overall well-being.

Strategies for Sugar Reduction

<u>Choose Whole Foods:</u>

Opt for whole, unprocessed foods whenever possible. Fruits, vegetables, lean proteins, and whole grains provide essential nutrients without added sugars.

<u>Cook at Home:</u>

Cooking meals from scratch gives you full control over ingredients, reducing the risk of hidden sugars sneaking into your diet.

<u>Swap Sugary Drinks:</u>

Replace sugary beverages like soda, fruit juices, and energy drinks with water, herbal teas, or sparkling water with a splash of lemon or lime.

<u>Read Recipes Carefully:</u>

When following recipes, scrutinize ingredient lists for hidden sugars. Look for healthier substitutes or consider reducing sugar amounts.

<u>Conclusion:</u>

Identifying hidden sugars is a vital aspect of managing diabetes through diet. By educating oneself on sugar sources, reading labels diligently, and making conscious food choices, individuals can take control of their health and mitigate the impact of sugar on blood sugar levels. Empowered with knowledge, individuals can navigate the modern food landscape with confidence, making informed decisions to support their diabetes management goals.

Making Informed Choices

In the realm of diabetes management, making informed choices is paramount to maintaining optimal health. From food selection to physical activity and medication management, every decision plays a role in controlling blood sugar levels and preventing complications. By understanding the principles of nutrition, exercise, and medication, individuals can empower themselves to make informed choices that support their journey towards better diabetes management.

Nutrition

Understanding Macronutrients:

Carbohydrates, proteins, and fats all affect blood sugar levels differently. Learning how to balance these macronutrients in meals can help stabilize blood sugar levels throughout the day.

Glycemic Index and Load:

Familiarizing oneself with the glycemic index (GI) and glycemic load (GL) of foods can aid in selecting options that have less impact on blood sugar levels. Foods with lower GI and GL values cause slower and steadier rises in blood sugar.

Portion Control: Managing portion sizes is crucial for regulating blood sugar levels. Measuring portions, using smaller plates, and paying attention to hunger and fullness cues can prevent overeating and blood sugar spikes.

Meal Planning: Planning meals ahead of time allows for better control over food choices and portion sizes. Creating balanced meals that include a variety of nutrient-rich foods can help maintain steady blood sugar levels throughout the day.

Exercise

<u>Importance of Physical Activity:</u>

Regular exercise helps improve insulin sensitivity, making it easier for cells to absorb glucose from the bloodstream. Aim for a combination of aerobic exercise, strength training, and flexibility exercises for overall health benefits.

<u>Setting Realistic Goals:</u> Establish achievable exercise goals based on individual fitness levels, preferences, and health status. Start with small, manageable goals and gradually increase intensity and duration over time.

<u>Incorporating Exercise into Daily Routine:</u> Finding opportunities to be active throughout the day can contribute to overall physical fitness. Simple activities like taking the stairs, walking or biking to work, and incorporating movement breaks during sedentary activities can add up to significant health benefits.

Medication Management

<u>Adhering to Medication Regimen:</u>

Consistency is key when it comes to taking diabetes medications as prescribed. Establishing a routine and setting reminders can help ensure medications are taken on time.

<u>Understanding Medication Effects:</u>

Educate yourself about how different diabetes medications work and their potential side effects. Communicate openly with healthcare providers about any concerns or difficulties experienced with medications.

Monitoring Blood Sugar Levels:

Regularly monitoring blood sugar levels provides valuable insights into how lifestyle choices, including diet, exercise, and medication, affect glucose levels. Use this information to make adjustments as needed to maintain target blood sugar ranges.

Conclusion:

Making informed choices is the cornerstone of effective diabetes management. By educating oneself about nutrition, exercise, and medication, individuals with diabetes can take an active role in their health and well-being. Empowered with knowledge and equipped with practical strategies, they can navigate the complexities of diabetes management with confidence, leading to better outcomes and improved quality of life.

Chapter 5: Weight Management and Diabetes

Importance of Weight Management

In the realm of diabetes management, weight management emerges as a cornerstone of holistic care. While diabetes demands attention to various aspects of one's lifestyle, the significance of maintaining a healthy weight cannot be overstated. Here's why weight management is pivotal in the context of diabetes:

Blood Glucose Regulation

Excess weight, particularly abdominal fat, significantly impacts insulin sensitivity. By shedding extra pounds through dietary modifications and regular exercise, individuals can enhance insulin sensitivity, facilitating better control over blood glucose levels.

Risk Reduction

Obesity amplifies the risk of developing type 2 diabetes and exacerbates complications in those already diagnosed. Effective weight management serves as a potent tool in reducing this risk and mitigating the severity of associated complications, including cardiovascular diseases, neuropathy, and nephropathy.

Medication Optimization

Achieving a healthy weight often translates into improved medication efficacy. With weight loss, individuals may require lower doses of medication, reducing the likelihood of side effects and enhancing treatment outcomes. Additionally, some individuals may even experience a reduced need for medication altogether.

Enhanced Energy and Vitality

Shedding excess weight can lead to increased energy levels and vitality. This surge in energy empowers individuals to engage in regular physical activity, further bolstering their diabetes management efforts and fostering an overall sense of well-being.

Psychological Well-being

Struggling with weight can take a toll on one's mental health, contributing to stress, anxiety, and depression. Effective weight management not only improves physical health but also cultivates a positive mindset, bolstering self-esteem and confidence.

In essence, weight management is a fundamental pillar of diabetes care. By prioritizing weight loss through a balanced diet, physical activity, and lifestyle modifications, individuals can exert significant control over their condition, reduce complications, and pave the way for a healthier, more fulfilling life.

Healthy Weight Loss Strategies

Achieving and maintaining a healthy weight is crucial for individuals with diabetes. However, embarking on a weight loss journey requires careful consideration of effective and sustainable strategies. Here are some healthy weight loss strategies tailored to individuals managing diabetes:

Balanced Diet

Adopting a balanced diet is paramount for sustainable weight loss and diabetes management. Focus on consuming whole, nutrient-dense foods such as fruits, vegetables, lean proteins, whole grains, and healthy fats. Incorporating fiber-rich foods can aid in satiety and blood sugar control.

Portion Control

Paying attention to portion sizes is key in managing calorie intake and promoting weight loss. Use measuring cups, food scales, or visual cues to gauge appropriate portion sizes. Avoid oversized servings, especially of high-calorie foods, to prevent excess calorie consumption.

Carbohydrate Management

Carbohydrates have a significant impact on blood sugar levels. Opt for complex carbohydrates with a low glycemic index, such as whole grains, legumes, and non-starchy vegetables. Distribute carbohydrate intake evenly throughout the day to prevent spikes in blood glucose levels.

Regular Physical Activity

Incorporating regular physical activity into your routine is essential for both weight loss and diabetes management. Aim for a combination of aerobic exercise, strength training, and flexibility exercises. Consult with a healthcare professional to develop a personalized exercise plan tailored to your needs and capabilities.

Mindful Eating

Practice mindful eating by paying attention to hunger cues, eating slowly, and savoring each bite. Avoid distractions such as screens or work during meals to promote awareness of food intake. This approach can prevent overeating and promote healthier food choices.

Hydration

Stay hydrated by drinking plenty of water throughout the day. Sometimes, thirst can be mistaken for hunger, leading to unnecessary snacking. Drinking water can help curb appetite and support weight loss efforts.

Stress Management

Chronic stress can interfere with weight loss efforts and exacerbate diabetes symptoms. Incorporate stress-reducing activities into your routine, such as meditation, yoga, deep breathing exercises, or spending time in nature. Prioritize self-care to promote overall well-being.

Regular Monitoring

Monitor your progress regularly by tracking food intake, physical activity, blood sugar levels, and weight. This allows you to identify patterns, make adjustments as needed, and celebrate successes along the way.

By adopting these healthy weight loss strategies, individuals with diabetes can achieve sustainable weight loss, improve blood sugar control, reduce the risk of complications, and enhance overall quality of life. Remember to consult with a healthcare professional before making significant changes to your diet or exercise regimen.

Exercise and Diabetes

Exercise is a cornerstone of diabetes management, offering a multitude of benefits that extend beyond physical fitness. In this section, we explore the profound impact of exercise on diabetes and provide practical insights for incorporating physical activity into daily life:

Blood Sugar Regulation

Regular physical activity enhances insulin sensitivity, enabling cells to better utilize glucose for energy. This helps to stabilize blood sugar levels, reducing the risk of hyperglycemia and hypoglycemia. Incorporating both aerobic exercise and resistance training into your routine can yield optimal results.

Weight Management

Exercise plays a pivotal role in achieving and maintaining a healthy weight, which is essential for diabetes management. By burning calories and building lean muscle mass, physical activity helps to reduce body fat and improve overall body composition. This, in turn, enhances insulin sensitivity and reduces the risk of obesity-related complications.

Cardiovascular Health

Diabetes is associated with an increased risk of cardiovascular disease. Regular exercise strengthens the heart, improves circulation, and lowers blood pressure and cholesterol levels, reducing the risk of heart disease and stroke. Engaging in aerobic activities such as walking, jogging, cycling, or swimming can significantly benefit cardiovascular health.

Stress Reduction

Managing stress is crucial for diabetes management, as stress can elevate blood sugar levels and interfere with insulin sensitivity. Exercise acts as a natural stress reliever, releasing endorphins that promote feelings of well-being and relaxation. Incorporating activities such as yoga, tai chi, or mindfulness-based exercises can further enhance stress management.

Improved Mood and Mental Health

Living with diabetes can be challenging, and individuals may experience heightened levels of anxiety, depression, or diabetes-related distress. Exercise has been shown to improve mood, reduce symptoms of depression, and enhance overall mental well-being. The sense of accomplishment and empowerment gained from regular physical activity can boost self-confidence and resilience.

Diabetes Complication Prevention

Exercise helps to reduce the risk of diabetes-related complications, including neuropathy, nephropathy, and retinopathy. By improving circulation, lowering blood pressure, and promoting overall vascular health, physical activity contributes to the prevention and management of these complications.

Practical Tips for Incorporating Exercise

Start slowly and gradually increase the duration and intensity of your workouts to avoid injury. Choose activities that you enjoy and that fit your lifestyle, whether it's walking, dancing, gardening, or playing sports. Aim for at least 150 minutes of moderate-intensity aerobic exercise per week, supplemented with strength training exercises two to three times per week.

By making exercise a regular part of your diabetes management plan, you can experience a multitude of benefits that contribute to improved health and well-being. Remember to consult with your healthcare team before starting any new exercise regimen, especially if you have pre-existing health conditions or concerns. With dedication and perseverance, exercise can be a powerful tool in the management of diabetes.

Achieving weight loss is a significant accomplishment, but the journey doesn't end there. Maintaining weight loss over the long term is essential for effective diabetes management and overall health. In this section, we delve into strategies for sustaining weight loss and preventing regain:

Lifestyle Modification

Sustainable weight loss hinges on adopting healthy lifestyle habits that promote long-term success. Focus on making gradual, sustainable changes to your diet and physical activity routine rather than resorting to short-term fad diets or extreme exercise regimens. Embrace a balanced diet rich in fruits, vegetables, lean proteins, and whole grains, and incorporate regular physical activity into your daily routine.

Regular Monitoring

Stay vigilant by regularly monitoring your weight, food intake, physical activity, and blood sugar levels. Keeping track of your progress allows you to identify any deviations from your plan early on and make necessary adjustments to stay on track. Consider keeping a food diary, using a fitness tracker, or scheduling regular check-ins with a healthcare professional for accountability and support.

Mindful Eating

Practice mindful eating by paying attention to hunger and satiety cues, eating slowly, and savoring each bite. Avoid distractions such as screens or work during meals to promote awareness of food intake. By cultivating a mindful approach to eating, you can prevent overeating, make healthier food choices, and maintain a healthy relationship with food.

Regular Physical Activity

Consistency is key when it comes to physical activity. Aim to incorporate regular exercise into your daily routine, choosing activities that you enjoy and that fit your lifestyle. Whether it's brisk walking, cycling, swimming, or yoga, find activities that you can sustain over the long term. Remember that even small bouts of activity add up and contribute to overall calorie expenditure.

Social Support

Surround yourself with a supportive network of friends, family members, or fellow individuals with diabetes who understand and encourage your weight loss journey. Joining a support group, attending fitness classes with friends, or seeking the guidance of a registered dietitian or certified diabetes educator can provide invaluable support and motivation along the way.

Flexibility and Adaptability

Life is full of challenges and setbacks, and maintaining weight loss is no exception. Be prepared to adapt to changes in your routine, environment, or circumstances that may impact your ability to stick to your plan. Rather than viewing setbacks as failures, approach them as opportunities to learn and grow, and recommit to your goals with renewed determination.

Self-Compassion

Be kind to yourself throughout your weight loss journey. Celebrate your successes, no matter how small, and acknowledge the progress you've made. Practice self-compassion and forgiveness when faced with setbacks or challenges, and remember that sustainable weight loss is a marathon, not a sprint.

By incorporating these strategies into your daily life, you can sustain weight loss over the long term and reap the numerous benefits for diabetes management and overall well-being. Stay committed, stay focused, and remember that you have the power to achieve lasting success in your journey toward better health.

Chapter 6: Nutrients and Diabetes

Vitamins and Minerals

Proper nutrition plays a crucial role in diabetes management, and ensuring adequate intake of essential vitamins and minerals is key to supporting overall health and well-being. In this section, we explore the vital role of various vitamins and minerals in diabetes care and provide practical insights for incorporating them into your diet:

Vitamin D

Known as the "sunshine vitamin," vitamin D plays a critical role in insulin sensitivity and blood sugar regulation. Low levels of vitamin D have been associated with an increased risk of type 2 diabetes and complications such as cardiovascular disease. Incorporate vitamin D-rich foods such as fatty fish, fortified dairy products, eggs, and fortified cereals into your diet, and aim for moderate sun exposure to support natural vitamin D synthesis.

Magnesium

Magnesium is involved in over 300 enzymatic reactions in the body, including those related to glucose metabolism and insulin action. Research suggests that magnesium deficiency may contribute to insulin resistance and increase the risk of type 2 diabetes. Include magnesium-rich foods such as leafy green vegetables, nuts, seeds, whole grains, and legumes in your diet to support optimal magnesium levels.

Calcium

Calcium is essential for bone health and may also play a role in insulin secretion and glucose metabolism. Adequate calcium intake has been associated with a reduced risk of type 2 diabetes. Incorporate calcium-rich foods such as dairy products, leafy green vegetables, fortified plant-based milks, and tofu into your diet to support bone health and overall metabolic health.

Vitamin B12

Vitamin B12 is involved in energy production, nerve function, and red blood cell formation. Individuals with diabetes may have an increased risk of vitamin B12 deficiency due to certain medications and dietary factors. Include vitamin B12-rich foods such as meat, fish, poultry, eggs, dairy products, and fortified cereals in your diet, or consider supplementation if needed.

Vitamin C

Vitamin C is a powerful antioxidant that helps protect against oxidative stress and inflammation, both of which are associated with diabetes complications. Additionally, vitamin C may improve endothelial function and reduce the risk of cardiovascular disease in individuals with diabetes. Incorporate vitamin C-rich foods such as citrus fruits, berries, kiwi, peppers, and broccoli into your diet to support overall health and immune function.

Zinc

Zinc is involved in numerous enzymatic reactions in the body, including insulin synthesis, secretion, and action. Low zinc levels have been associated with impaired glucose metabolism and increased risk of diabetes complications. Include zinc-rich foods such as oysters, beef, poultry, nuts, seeds, and whole grains in your diet to support optimal zinc levels.

Potassium

Potassium plays a crucial role in regulating blood pressure, nerve function, and muscle contractions. Individuals with diabetes are at an increased risk of potassium deficiency due to certain medications and kidney disease. Include potassium-rich foods such as bananas, oranges, potatoes, spinach, and yogurt in your diet to support heart health and overall metabolic function.

By prioritizing a balanced diet rich in these essential vitamins and minerals, individuals with diabetes can support optimal health, manage blood sugar levels, and reduce the risk of complications. Remember to consult with a healthcare professional or registered dietitian for personalized guidance on meeting your nutrient needs and optimizing your diet for diabetes management.

Fiber and Diabetes

Fiber is a nutrient often overlooked but holds significant importance in the management of diabetes. In this section, we delve into the role of fiber in diabetes care and provide practical insights for incorporating fiber-rich foods into a balanced diet:

Blood Sugar Regulation

Fiber plays a pivotal role in regulating blood sugar levels by slowing down the absorption of glucose into the bloodstream. Soluble fiber, found in foods such as oats, legumes, fruits, and vegetables, forms a gel-like substance in the digestive tract, which helps to stabilize blood sugar levels and prevent spikes after meals. This can be particularly beneficial for individuals with diabetes in managing glycemic control.

Improved Insulin Sensitivity

Research suggests that diets rich in fiber may improve insulin sensitivity, making it easier for cells to respond to insulin and regulate blood sugar levels effectively. By incorporating fiber-rich foods into your diet, you can support optimal insulin function and reduce the risk of insulin resistance, a hallmark of type 2 diabetes.

Weight Management

Fiber-rich foods tend to be low in calories and high in volume, which can promote feelings of fullness and satiety. By including more fiber in your diet, you can curb hunger cravings, reduce calorie intake, and support weight management efforts. This is particularly important for individuals with diabetes, as maintaining a healthy weight is key to managing the condition effectively.

Digestive Health

Fiber is essential for maintaining digestive health and preventing constipation. Insoluble fiber, found in foods such as whole grains, nuts, seeds, and vegetables, adds bulk to stool and promotes regularity. By supporting digestive health, fiber can help individuals with diabetes manage common gastrointestinal issues and improve overall well-being.

Heart Health Benefits

Fiber-rich diets have been associated with a reduced risk of heart disease, a common complication of diabetes. Soluble fiber helps to lower LDL (bad) cholesterol levels by binding to cholesterol particles and promoting their excretion from the body. By lowering cholesterol levels and improving heart health, fiber can reduce the risk of cardiovascular events in individuals with diabetes.

Practical Tips for Increasing Fiber Intake Incorporating more fiber into your diet is easier than you might think. Start by including a variety of fiber-rich foods such as fruits, vegetables, whole grains, legumes, nuts, and seeds in your meals and snacks. Aim to fill half your plate with non-starchy vegetables, choose whole grains over refined grains, and snack on fruits or raw vegetables instead of processed snacks. Gradually increase your fiber intake to avoid digestive discomfort, and remember to drink plenty of water to help fiber move through the digestive tract smoothly.

By prioritizing fiber-rich foods in your diet, you can reap numerous benefits for diabetes management, including better blood sugar control, improved insulin sensitivity, weight management support, digestive health promotion, and reduced risk of heart disease. Embrace the power of fiber as part of a balanced eating plan for optimal health and well-being.

The Role of Antioxidants

Antioxidants are compounds found in foods that help neutralize harmful molecules called free radicals, which can damage cells and contribute to chronic diseases, including diabetes. In this section, we explore the vital role of antioxidants in diabetes care and provide practical insights for incorporating antioxidant-rich foods into a balanced diet:

Protection Against Oxidative Stress

Individuals with diabetes are particularly susceptible to oxidative stress, a condition characterized by an imbalance between free radicals and antioxidants in the body. Excess glucose in the bloodstream can promote the production of free radicals, leading to cellular damage and inflammation. Antioxidants help counteract this oxidative damage, protecting cells from harm and reducing the risk of diabetes-related complications.

Improved Blood Sugar Control

Some antioxidants have been shown to improve blood sugar control and insulin sensitivity in individuals with diabetes. For example, polyphenols found in foods such as berries, dark chocolate, and green tea may help regulate blood glucose levels by enhancing insulin secretion and reducing insulin resistance. By incorporating antioxidant-rich foods into your diet, you can support better glycemic control and reduce the risk of hyperglycemia and hypoglycemia.

Heart Health Benefits

Diabetes is a major risk factor for cardiovascular disease, and protecting heart health is paramount for individuals with diabetes. Antioxidants, particularly flavonoids found in fruits, vegetables, and whole grains, have been associated with a reduced risk of heart disease by lowering blood pressure, improving blood vessel function, and reducing inflammation. By consuming a diet rich in antioxidants, you can support cardiovascular health and reduce the risk of heart-related complications.

Anti-inflammatory Properties

Chronic inflammation is a common feature of diabetes and is linked to the development of insulin resistance and complications such as heart disease and kidney disease. Antioxidants help combat inflammation by neutralizing inflammatory molecules and reducing the production of pro-inflammatory substances. Foods rich in antioxidants, such as colorful fruits and vegetables, nuts, seeds, and spices, can help quell inflammation and promote overall health.

Eye Health Protection

Diabetes can increase the risk of diabetic retinopathy, a leading cause of blindness in adults. Antioxidants such as vitamins C and E, lutein, and zeaxanthin have been shown to protect against eye damage by reducing oxidative stress and inflammation in the retina. Including antioxidant-rich foods in your diet may help preserve vision and reduce the risk of diabetic eye complications.

Practical Tips for Increasing Antioxidant Intake

Incorporating more antioxidant-rich foods into your diet is simple and delicious. Focus on consuming a variety of colorful fruits and vegetables, as vibrant hues often indicate high antioxidant content. Berries, citrus fruits, leafy greens, tomatoes, bell peppers, and broccoli are excellent sources of antioxidants. Additionally, include nuts, seeds, whole grains, and herbs and spices such as turmeric, cinnamon, and ginger in your meals and snacks to boost antioxidant intake.

By embracing a diet rich in antioxidants, individuals with diabetes can harness the power of these potent compounds to support better blood sugar control, protect against complications, and promote overall health and well-being. Make antioxidant-rich foods a central part of your eating plan to nourish your body and optimize diabetes management.

Hydration and Diabetes

Hydration is pivotal in diabetes management, impacting various facets of health. Here, we delve into its significance and offer practical tips for maintaining optimal hydration:

Blood Sugar Balance

Adequate hydration aids in blood sugar regulation. Dehydration can elevate blood glucose levels, complicating diabetes management. Proper hydration supports kidney function, assisting in the removal of excess glucose through urine. Consistently drinking water throughout the day helps maintain stable blood sugar levels.

Kidney Function Support

Diabetes increases the risk of kidney complications. Hydration is vital for kidney health, as it enables efficient filtration of waste products and toxins. Proper hydration reduces the strain on the kidneys, minimizing the risk of diabetic nephropathy. It's essential to strike a balance, as excessive fluid intake can strain the kidneys, particularly in individuals with kidney disease.

Preventing Dehydration-Related Complications

Dehydration poses risks for individuals with diabetes, such as diabetic ketoacidosis (DKA). DKA occurs when insulin deficiency leads to the body breaking down fat for energy, resulting in ketone production and acidosis. Adequate hydration helps prevent DKA by supporting insulin function and facilitating glucose utilization.

Promoting Cardiovascular Health

Diabetes increases the risk of cardiovascular disease. Proper hydration supports heart health by maintaining blood volume and circulation. It helps prevent complications like hypertension and reduces the risk of heart attacks and strokes. Drinking water regularly supports overall cardiovascular well-being.

Enhancing Exercise Performance

Physical activity is crucial for diabetes management, but dehydration can impair exercise performance. Proper hydration ensures optimal muscle function and endurance during workouts. It's essential to hydrate before, during, and after exercise, particularly in hot or humid conditions.

Practical Hydration Tips

Aim to drink water consistently throughout the day, even if you're not thirsty. Carry a reusable water bottle to encourage hydration. Monitor urine color—pale yellow indicates adequate hydration, while darker urine suggests the need for more fluids. Limit intake of sugary or caffeinated beverages, as they can contribute to dehydration. Hydration requirements vary based on factors such as age, weight, activity level, climate, and health status. Individuals with diabetes should consult healthcare providers to determine personalized hydration goals and strategies.

In conclusion, maintaining proper hydration is essential for individuals with diabetes. By prioritizing hydration as part of a comprehensive diabetes management plan, individuals can support blood sugar control, kidney health, cardiovascular function, and overall well-being.

Chapter 7: Diabetes and Eating Disorders

Recognizing Eating Disorders

Eating disorders can significantly impact the physical and mental health of individuals with diabetes, complicating diabetes management and increasing the risk of serious health consequences. In this section, we explore the importance of recognizing eating disorders in individuals with diabetes and provide guidance on how to identify warning signs:

Understanding the Link

The intersection of diabetes and eating disorders is complex. For some individuals, the emphasis on food, weight, and body image management inherent in diabetes self-care can trigger disordered eating behaviors. Others may develop eating disorders independently of their diabetes diagnosis. It's essential to recognize the interplay between these conditions and address them comprehensively.

Common Eating Disorders

Several eating disorders commonly co-occur with diabetes, including:

Binge Eating Disorder (BED):
Characterized by recurrent episodes of uncontrollable eating, often resulting in feelings of guilt, shame, and distress.

<u>Anorexia Nervosa:</u> Involves severe restriction of food intake, fear of gaining weight, and distorted body image.

<u>Bulimia Nervosa:</u> Involves episodes of binge eating followed by compensatory behaviors such as vomiting, excessive exercise, or misuse of insulin or other diabetes medications to control weight.

Warning Signs:

Recognizing the warning signs of eating disorders in individuals with diabetes is crucial for early intervention. These may include:

-Obsessive preoccupation with food, weight, and body image.

-Extreme fluctuations in weight or blood sugar levels.

-Secretive eating behaviors, such as eating alone or in isolation.

-Excessive concern about the nutritional content or calorie   count of foods.

-Avoidance of social situations involving food.

-Frequent use of laxatives, diuretics, or insulin manipulation for weight control.

Impact on Diabetes Management

Eating disorders can have serious consequences for diabetes management, leading to erratic blood sugar levels, insulin misuse, and poor adherence to treatment regimens. Individuals with diabetes and eating disorders are at increased risk of diabetic ketoacidosis, hypoglycemia, and long-term complications such as retinopathy, neuropathy, and cardiovascular disease.

Seeking Support

If you suspect that you or someone you know is struggling with an eating disorder, it's essential to seek help promptly. Consult with a healthcare professional, such as a primary care physician, endocrinologist, or mental health specialist, who can provide a comprehensive assessment and recommend appropriate treatment options. Treatment typically involves a multidisciplinary approach, including medical management, nutritional counseling, psychotherapy, and support groups.

Promoting Positive Body Image

Encourage individuals with diabetes to cultivate a positive body image and practice self-compassion. Emphasize the importance of self-care and self-acceptance, regardless of weight or physical appearance. Encourage healthy behaviors, such as engaging in enjoyable physical activities, prioritizing balanced nutrition, and seeking social support.

By recognizing the signs of eating disorders in individuals with diabetes and providing timely intervention and support, we can help promote better health outcomes and improved quality of life for those affected by these challenging conditions. It's essential to approach the topic with empathy, understanding, and a commitment to holistic care.

Diabulimia: The Dangerous Combination

Diabulimia is a term used to describe the dangerous practice of individuals with Type 1 diabetes intentionally restricting their insulin intake to lose weight. It's a harmful combination of diabetes management and eating disorder behaviors that can have severe consequences on both physical and mental health.

The Dangers of Diabulimia

<u>Uncontrolled Blood Sugar Levels:</u>

Insulin is essential for regulating blood sugar levels. Without enough insulin, glucose builds up in the bloodstream, leading to hyperglycemia, which can cause short-term symptoms like frequent urination, thirst, and fatigue, as well as long-term complications such as nerve damage, kidney failure, and vision problems.

<u>Increased Risk of Diabetic Ketoacidosis (DKA):</u> DKA is a serious condition that occurs when the body doesn't have enough insulin and begins to break down fat for energy, producing toxic ketones as a byproduct. Diabulimia significantly increases the risk of DKA, which can be life-threatening if not treated promptly.

<u>Nutritional Deficiencies:</u>

Skipping insulin to manipulate weight can lead to inadequate nutrient absorption, resulting in deficiencies in essential vitamins and minerals. This can weaken the immune system, impair organ function, and hinder overall health.

<u>Negative Impact on Mental Health:</u>

Diabulimia is not just a physical health concern; it also takes a toll on mental well-being. The constant cycle of disordered eating behaviors, guilt, and shame can contribute to anxiety, depression, and other psychological issues.

<u>Increased Mortality Risk:</u>

Studies have shown that individuals with Type 1 diabetes who engage in diabulimia have a significantly higher mortality rate compared to those who don't. The combination of diabetes complications and the effects of an eating disorder can have devastating consequences.

Treatment and Prevention

<u>Education and Awareness:</u>

Healthcare providers need to be trained to recognize the signs of diabulimia and provide appropriate support and treatment. Similarly, individuals with diabetes should be educated about the risks of manipulating insulin for weight loss and the importance of seeking help if they're struggling.

<u>Integrated Care:</u>

Treatment for diabulimia requires a multidisciplinary approach that addresses both the physical and psychological aspects of the disorder. This may include medical monitoring, nutritional counseling, therapy (such as cognitive-behavioral therapy), and support groups.

<u>Body Positivity and Acceptance:</u>

Promoting body positivity and self-acceptance can help combat the societal pressures to attain unrealistic body standards. Encouraging individuals to focus on overall health and well-being rather than just weight can reduce the likelihood of developing harmful behaviors like diabulimia.

Diabulimia is a dangerous combination of diabetes and eating disorder behaviors that poses significant risks to both physical and mental health. By raising awareness, providing appropriate support and treatment, and promoting body positivity, we can work towards preventing and addressing this harmful phenomenon.

Support and Resources

Dealing with both diabetes and eating disorders can present unique challenges, but there are numerous support systems and resources available to help you navigate these complex conditions. Here are some valuable avenues to explore:

Specialized Treatment Centers

Look for treatment centers or clinics that specialize in treating individuals with co-occurring diabetes and eating disorders. These facilities offer comprehensive care from multidisciplinary teams of healthcare professionals, including doctors, therapists, dietitians, and diabetes educators.

Therapy and Counseling

Individual therapy or counseling sessions with a psychologist or therapist who specializes in eating disorders and/or diabetes management can provide invaluable support. Cognitive-behavioral therapy (CBT), dialectical behavior therapy (DBT), and acceptance and commitment therapy (ACT) are often effective in addressing the underlying emotional and behavioral aspects of these conditions.

Support Groups

Joining a support group specifically tailored to individuals with diabetes and eating disorders can offer a sense of community, understanding, and encouragement. These groups provide a safe space to share experiences, receive peer support, and learn coping strategies for managing both conditions simultaneously.

Online Communities

Participating in online forums, chat rooms, or social media groups dedicated to diabetes and eating disorders can connect you with others who are going through similar experiences. These virtual communities offer support, validation, and practical advice from individuals who understand the unique challenges of balancing diabetes management with recovery from an eating disorder.

Registered Dietitians

Collaborate with a registered dietitian who has experience working with individuals with diabetes and eating disorders. They can help you develop a balanced meal plan that supports both your diabetes management goals and your recovery from disordered eating behaviors. A dietitian can also provide education on intuitive eating, mindful eating, and body acceptance.

Medical Monitoring

Regular medical monitoring is essential for individuals with diabetes and eating disorders to ensure their physical health and safety. Work closely with your healthcare team, including your primary care physician, endocrinologist, and mental health professionals, to monitor your blood sugar levels, nutritional status, and overall well-being.

Educational Resources

Educate yourself about the relationship between diabetes and eating disorders through books, articles, and online resources. The National Eating Disorders Association (NEDA) and the American Diabetes Association (ADA) offer educational materials, webinars, and online courses that address the intersection of these conditions.

Self-Care Practices

Practice self-care strategies to support your overall well-being and manage stress. Engage in activities that promote relaxation, such as mindfulness meditation, yoga, or journaling. Prioritize adequate sleep, regular physical activity, and healthy coping mechanisms to maintain balance in your life.

Remember, seeking help and support is a courageous step towards healing and recovery. You are not alone, and there are people and resources available to support you on your journey towards better health and well-being. Don't hesitate to reach out for help when you need it.

Chapter 8: Diabetes Myths and Facts

Debunking Common Myths

Here are some common myths about diabetes along with why they should be taken with a grain of salt.

Myth 1: Eating too much sugar causes diabetes.

<u>Fact</u>: While consuming excessive sugar isn't good for overall health, it doesn't directly cause diabetes. Type 1 diabetes is an autoimmune condition, and type 2 diabetes is influenced by various factors including genetics, lifestyle, and weight.

Myth 2: People with diabetes can't eat carbohydrates.

<u>Fact</u>: Carbohydrates are part of a balanced diet and can be included in moderation. The key is to choose healthy carbohydrates like whole grains, fruits, and vegetables, and to monitor portion sizes.

Myth 3: Only overweight or obese people get diabetes.

<u>Fact</u>: While being overweight or obese increases the risk of type 2 diabetes, it's not the only factor. Thin people can also develop diabetes, especially type 1 diabetes which is not related to weight.

Myth 4: Insulin is a cure for diabetes.

<u>Fact</u>: Insulin is a treatment for diabetes, not a cure. It helps manage blood sugar levels, but it doesn't eliminate the underlying causes of diabetes. Lifestyle changes such as diet and exercise are also important in managing diabetes.

Myth 5: Diabetes is not a serious disease.

<u>Fact</u>: Diabetes can lead to serious complications such as heart disease, stroke, kidney disease, and vision problems if not properly managed. It requires careful monitoring and management to prevent complications and maintain overall health.

Myth 6: People with diabetes can't lead a normal life.

<u>Fact</u>: With proper management, people with diabetes can lead full and active lives. This includes monitoring blood sugar levels, taking medication as prescribed, eating a balanced diet, exercising regularly, and attending regular medical check-ups.

By addressing these myths, readers can gain a better understanding of diabetes and make informed decisions about their diet and lifestyle.

Understanding the Facts

Now that we've debunked some common myths surrounding diabetes, let's delve into the key facts you need to know about this condition:

Types of Diabetes

Diabetes is not a one-size-fits-all condition. There are primarily two main types:

Type 1 Diabetes

Type 2 Diabetes

The explanation for what exactly these are, is stated earlier in the book.

Blood Sugar Management

One of the primary goals in managing diabetes is to keep blood sugar levels within a target range. This requires a combination of medication (such as insulin or oral medications), dietary modifications, regular physical activity, and monitoring blood sugar levels.

Importance of Diet

Diet plays a crucial role in managing diabetes. While there's no one-size-fits-all approach, a balanced diet rich in whole grains, fruits, vegetables, lean proteins, and healthy fats is recommended. Monitoring carbohydrate intake, portion sizes, and spacing meals evenly throughout the day can help stabilize blood sugar levels.

Physical Activity

Regular exercise is beneficial for everyone, but it's especially important for people with diabetes. Physical activity helps lower blood sugar levels, improve insulin sensitivity, manage weight, reduce the risk of heart disease, and enhance overall well-being. Aim for at least 150 minutes of moderate-intensity aerobic activity per week, along with strength training exercises at least twice a week.

Monitoring and Management

Monitoring blood sugar levels regularly is essential for managing diabetes effectively. This may involve self-monitoring using a blood glucose meter or continuous glucose monitoring (CGM) system. Additionally, regular medical check-ups, including A1C tests, lipid profiles, and kidney function tests, are crucial for assessing overall health and detecting any complications early.

By understanding these facts about diabetes, you can empower yourself to make informed decisions about your diet, lifestyle, and overall health management. Remember, knowledge is key to effectively managing diabetes and living a fulfilling life.

The Truth about Sugar and Diabetes

Sugar often gets a bad rap when it comes to diabetes, but let's uncover the truth about its role in managing this condition:

Understanding Sugar

Sugars are carbohydrates found naturally in foods such as fruits, vegetables, dairy products, and grains. They also include added sugars found in sweets, sodas, processed foods, and sugary beverages.

Effect on Blood Sugar

All carbohydrates, including sugars, can affect blood sugar levels. When you consume sugary foods or beverages, your blood sugar may rise more quickly compared to when you consume complex carbohydrates like whole grains or vegetables. However, it's not just sugar that affects blood sugar levels; the total amount of carbohydrates consumed and how they're balanced with other nutrients play a significant role.

Moderation is Key

Contrary to popular belief, you don't have to completely eliminate sugar from your diet if you have diabetes. Instead, focus on moderation and portion control. It's essential to be mindful of your total carbohydrate intake and how it fits into your overall meal plan. Choose healthier sources of carbohydrates such as whole fruits, which also provide fiber and essential nutrients.

Sugar and Type 2 Diabetes

While consuming excessive amounts of sugary foods and beverages can contribute to weight gain, which is a risk factor for type 2 diabetes, sugar alone is not the sole culprit. Type 2 diabetes is a complex condition influenced by various factors, including genetics, lifestyle, and overall dietary patterns.

Sugar and Type 1 Diabetes

For people with type 1 diabetes who require insulin injections to manage their condition, it's important to understand how different foods, including those containing sugar, can affect blood sugar levels. Consistent carbohydrate counting and insulin management are key strategies for maintaining stable blood sugar levels while still enjoying a variety of foods, including those with sugar.

Reading Labels

When selecting packaged foods, reading nutrition labels can help you make informed choices about sugar content. Keep an eye out for hidden sugars under various names such as sucrose, fructose, glucose, corn syrup, and maltose. Pay attention to portion sizes and aim for products with lower added sugar content.

By understanding the truth about sugar and its relationship to diabetes, you can make empowered choices about your diet while still enjoying the foods you love in moderation. Remember, it's all about balance and moderation when it comes to managing diabetes effectively.

Fact-checking Diabetic Diets

Navigating dietary choices can be overwhelming, especially when it comes to managing diabetes. So Let's debunk more myths!

Myth 1: All sugars are off-limits for people with diabetes

<u>Fact:</u> While it's important to moderate intake of added sugars and sugary beverages, natural sugars found in whole foods like fruits and dairy products can be part of a balanced diabetic diet. These foods also

provide essential nutrients and fiber, which can help manage blood sugar levels.

Myth 2: Diabetic-friendly foods are always healthier.

<u>Fact:</u> Many "diabetic-friendly" foods marketed as sugar-free or low-carb may still contain unhealthy ingredients like artificial sweeteners, refined grains, and trans fats. Instead of relying on processed "diabetic" products, focus on whole, nutrient-dense foods like lean proteins, healthy fats, and high-fiber carbohydrates.

Myth 3: Eating small, frequent meals is necessary for diabetes management.

<u>Fact:</u> While some people with diabetes may benefit from spacing out meals to help manage blood sugar levels, others may find success with three balanced meals per day. The key is to find a meal pattern that works for your body and lifestyle while maintaining consistent carbohydrate intake throughout the day.

Myth 4: A diabetic diet means sacrificing taste and variety.

<u>Fact:</u> Managing diabetes doesn't mean giving up delicious foods or culinary creativity. There are countless flavorful recipes and meal ideas that align with a diabetic-friendly diet. Experiment with herbs, spices, and healthy cooking techniques to enhance the taste of your meals without compromising on nutrition.

Myth: Alcohol is completely off-limits for people with diabetes.

<u>Fact:</u> Moderate alcohol consumption may be acceptable for some people with diabetes, but it's essential to be mindful of its effects on blood sugar levels and overall health. Limit alcohol intake to no more than one drink per day for women and two drinks per day for men, and always consume it with food to help prevent low blood sugar.

By fact-checking common beliefs about the diabetic diet, you can make informed choices that support your overall health and well-being. Remember, there's no one-size-fits-all approach to nutrition, so work with a healthcare professional to develop a personalized eating plan that meets your special needs.

Chapter 9: Diabetic-Friendly Recipes

Breakfast Recipes

Vegetable Omelette

Ingredients:

- 2 eggs
- 1/4 cup diced bell peppers
- 1/4 cup diced tomatoes
- 1/4 cup diced onions
- 1/4 cup chopped spinach
- Salt and pepper to taste
- 1 teaspoon olive oil

Instructions:

1. In a bowl, beat the eggs and season with salt and pepper.

2. Heat olive oil in a non-stick skillet over medium heat.

3. Add the diced vegetables and sauté until tender.

4. Pour the beaten eggs over the vegetables in the skillet.

5. Cook until the eggs are set and the bottom is golden brown, then fold the omelette in half.

6. Serve hot with a side of whole grain toast or fresh fruit.

Greek Yogurt Parfait

Ingredients:

- 1/2 cup plain Greek yogurt

- 1/4 cup fresh berries (such as strawberries, blueberries, or raspberries)

- 1 tablespoon chopped nuts (such as almonds or walnuts)

- 1 tablespoon ground flaxseeds

- 1 teaspoon honey (optional)

<u>Instructions:</u>

1. In a glass or bowl, layer the Greek yogurt, fresh berries, chopped nuts, and ground flaxseeds.

2. Drizzle with honey if desired for added sweetness.

3. Serve immediately as a nutritious and satisfying breakfast option.

Whole Grain Pancakes

<u>Ingredients:</u>

- 1/2 cup whole wheat flour

- 1/4 cup oat flour

- 1 teaspoon baking powder

- 1/2 teaspoon cinnamon

- 1/2 cup unsweetened almond milk (or milk of choice)

- 1 egg

- 1 tablespoon unsweetened applesauce

- 1 teaspoon vanilla extract

- Cooking spray

<u>Instructions:</u>

1. In a mixing bowl, combine the whole wheat flour, oat flour, baking powder, and cinnamon.

2. In a separate bowl, whisk together the almond milk, egg, applesauce, and vanilla extract.

3. Pour the wet ingredients into the dry ingredients and stir until well combined.

4. Heat a non-stick skillet over medium heat and lightly coat with cooking spray.

5. Pour 1/4 cup of batter onto the skillet for each pancake.

6. Cook until bubbles form on the surface, then flip and cook until golden brown on both sides.

7. Serve warm with a dollop of Greek yogurt and fresh fruit.

These diabetic-friendly breakfast recipes are not only delicious but also nutritious, providing a balance of carbohydrates, protein, and fiber to help stabilize blood sugar levels throughout the morning.

Lunch Recipes

Here are some diabetic-friendly lunch recipes you can try.

Quinoa Salad with Chickpeas and Vegetables

Ingredients:

- 1 cup cooked quinoa
- 1/2 cup cooked chickpeas (canned, drained, and rinsed)
- 1/2 cup diced cucumber
- 1/2 cup diced bell peppers

- 1/4 cup diced red onion

- 1/4 cup chopped fresh parsley

- 2 tablespoons extra virgin olive oil

- 1 tablespoon lemon juice

- Salt and pepper to taste

Instructions:

1. In a large mixing bowl, combine the cooked quinoa, chickpeas, cucumber, bell peppers, red onion, and parsley.

2. In a small bowl, whisk together the olive oil, lemon juice, salt, and pepper to make the dressing.

3. Pour the dressing over the quinoa salad and toss until well combined.

4. Serve chilled or at room temperature as a satisfying and nutritious lunch option.

Grilled Chicken Wrap

Ingredients:

- 1 whole wheat or spinach tortilla

- 3 ounces grilled chicken breast, sliced

- 1/4 avocado, sliced

- 1/4 cup shredded lettuce

- 2 tablespoons diced tomatoes

- 1 tablespoon plain Greek yogurt (optional)

Instructions:

1. Lay the tortilla flat on a clean surface.

2. Layer the grilled chicken slices, avocado slices, shredded lettuce, and diced tomatoes in the center of the tortilla.

3. If desired, spread a tablespoon of plain Greek yogurt over the filling for added creaminess.

4. Fold the sides of the tortilla over the filling, then roll it up tightly from the bottom to form a wrap.

5. Slice the wrap in half diagonally and serve immediately, or wrap it tightly in foil or parchment paper for later.

Mediterranean Lentil Soup

Ingredients:

- 1 tablespoon olive oil
- 1/2 cup diced onion
- 2 cloves garlic, minced
- 1 carrot, diced
- 1 celery stalk, diced
- 1/2 cup dried green lentils, rinsed and drained
- 4 cups low-sodium vegetable broth
- 1 can (14.5 ounces) diced tomatoes, with juices
- 1 teaspoon dried oregano
- 1 teaspoon dried basil
- Salt and pepper to taste

Instructions:

1. Heat olive oil in a large pot over medium heat. Add the diced onion and garlic, and sauté until fragrant.

2. Add the diced carrot and celery to the pot, and cook for another 2-3 minutes.

3. Stir in the rinsed lentils, vegetable broth, diced tomatoes (with juices), oregano, basil, salt, and pepper.

4. Bring the soup to a boil, then reduce heat to low and let it simmer for about 25-30 minutes, or until the lentils are tender.

5. Taste and adjust seasoning if necessary. Serve hot, garnished with fresh parsley if desired.

These diabetic-friendly lunch recipes are not only delicious and satisfying but also provide a balance of nutrients to help keep blood sugar levels stable throughout the day.

Dinner Recipes

Baked Salmon with Roasted Vegetables

Ingredients:

- 4 salmon fillets (about 4 ounces each)

- 2 tablespoons olive oil

- 1 teaspoon dried thyme

- 1 teaspoon dried rosemary

- Salt and pepper to taste

- 2 cups mixed vegetables (such as bell peppers, zucchini, and cherry tomatoes), chopped

- 1 tablespoon balsamic vinegar

Instructions:

1. Pre heat the oven to 400°F (200°C). Line a baking sheet with parchment paper.

2. Place the salmon fillets on the prepared baking sheet. Drizzle with olive oil and sprinkle with dried thyme, dried rosemary, salt, and pepper.

3. In a bowl, toss the mixed vegetables with olive oil, balsamic vinegar, salt, and pepper. Spread them around the salmon on the baking sheet.

4. Bake in the preheated oven for 12-15 minutes, or until the salmon is cooked through and the vegetables are tender.

5. Serve the baked salmon and roasted vegetables hot, garnished with fresh herbs if desired.

Turkey and Vegetable Stir-Fry

Ingredients:

- 1 tablespoon olive oil

- 1 pound lean ground turkey

- 2 cloves garlic, minced

- 1 teaspoon grated ginger

- 2 cups mixed vegetables (such as bell peppers, broccoli, and snap peas), sliced

- 2 tablespoons low-sodium soy sauce

- 1 tablespoon rice vinegar

- 1 teaspoon honey or maple syrup

- Cooked brown rice or quinoa for serving

Instructions:

1. Heat olive oil in a large skillet or wok over medium-high heat. Add the ground turkey and cook until browned, breaking it apart with a spatula.

2. Add the minced garlic and grated ginger to the skillet, and cook for another minute until fragrant.

3. Stir in the mixed vegetables and cook until they are tender-crisp, about 5-7 minutes.

4. In a small bowl, whisk together the soy sauce, rice vinegar, and honey or maple syrup. Pour the sauce over the turkey and vegetables in the skillet, and toss to coat evenly.

5. Cook for an additional 2-3 minutes, then remove from heat.

6. Serve the turkey and vegetable stir-fry hot over cooked brown rice or quinoa.

Vegetarian Stuffed Bell Peppers

<u>Ingredients:</u>

- 4 large bell peppers, halved and seeds removed
- 1 cup cooked quinoa or brown rice
- 1 can (15 ounces) black beans, drained and rinsed
- 1 cup diced tomatoes
- 1/2 cup corn kernels
- 1/2 cup diced red onion
- 1 teaspoon chili powder
- 1/2 teaspoon cumin
- Salt and pepper to taste
- 1/2 cup shredded cheese (optional)

<u>Instructions:</u>

1. Preheat the oven to 375°F (190°C). Arrange the bell pepper halves in a baking dish.

2. In a large bowl, combine the cooked quinoa or brown rice, black beans, diced tomatoes, corn kernels, diced red onion, chili powder, cumin, salt, and pepper.

3. Spoon the quinoa and black bean mixture evenly into the bell pepper halves.

4. If desired, sprinkle shredded cheese on top of each stuffed pepper.

5. Cover the baking dish with foil and bake in the preheated oven for 25-30 minutes, or until the peppers are tender.

6. Remove the foil and bake for an additional 5 minutes to melt the cheese (if using).

7. Serve the vegetarian stuffed bell peppers hot, garnished with fresh cilantro or parsley if desired.

These diabetic-friendly dinner recipes are not only nutritious and delicious but also easy to prepare, making them perfect for busy weeknights.

Snack and Dessert Recipes

Apple Cinnamon Oatmeal Muffins

<u>Ingredients:</u>

- 1 cup rolled oats
- 1 cup whole wheat flour
- 1 teaspoon baking powder
- 1/2 teaspoon baking soda
- 1 teaspoon ground cinnamon
- 1/4 teaspoon salt
- 1/4 cup unsweetened applesauce
- 1/4 cup maple syrup or honey
- 1/4 cup plain Greek yogurt
- 1/4 cup milk of choice
- 1 egg
- 1 teaspoon vanilla extract
- 1 cup diced apples (about 1 medium apple)

1. Preheat the oven to 375°F (190°C). Line a muffin tin with paper liners or coat with non-stick cooking spray.

2. In a large bowl, combine the rolled oats, whole wheat flour, baking powder, baking soda, ground cinnamon, and salt.

3. In a separate bowl, whisk together the applesauce, maple syrup or honey, Greek yogurt, milk, egg, and vanilla extract until well combined.

4. Pour the wet ingredients into the dry ingredients and stir until just combined. Fold in the diced apples.

5. Divide the batter evenly among the prepared muffin cups, filling each about two-thirds full.

6. Bake in the preheated oven for 15-18 minutes, or until a toothpick inserted into the center of a muffin comes out clean.

7. Allow the muffins to cool in the pan for 5 minutes, then transfer them to a wire rack to cool completely.

8. Enjoy these delicious apple cinnamon oatmeal muffins as a wholesome snack or on-the-go breakfast option.

Greek Yogurt Berry Parfait

Ingredients:

- 1/2 cup plain Greek yogurt

- 1/4 cup mixed berries (such as strawberries, blueberries, and raspberries)

- 1 tablespoon chopped nuts (such as almonds or walnuts)

- 1 tablespoon unsweetened coconut flakes (optional)

- Drizzle of honey or maple syrup (optional)

Instructions:

1. In a glass or bowl, layer the plain Greek yogurt, mixed berries, chopped nuts, and coconut flakes.

2. Drizzle with honey or maple syrup if desired for added sweetness.

3. Serve immediately as a refreshing and nutritious snack or dessert option.

Dark Chocolate Covered Almonds

<u>Ingredients:</u>

- 1/2 cup raw almonds

- 2 ounces dark chocolate (at least 70% cocoa), chopped

- Pinch of sea salt

<u>Instructions:</u>

1. Line a baking sheet with parchment paper.

2. In a microwave-safe bowl, melt the dark chocolate in 30-second intervals, stirring in between, until smooth and melted.

3. Dip each almond into the melted chocolate, coating it evenly, then place it onto the prepared baking sheet.

4. Sprinkle a pinch of sea salt over the chocolate-covered almonds.

5. Allow the chocolate to set at room temperature or refrigerate for faster setting.

6. Once the chocolate is set, transfer the chocolate-covered almonds to an airtight container for storage.

7. Enjoy these indulgent dark chocolate covered almonds as a satisfying snack or dessert option in moderation.

These diabetic-friendly snack and dessert recipes are not only delicious but also provide a balance of nutrients to help satisfy your cravings without spiking blood sugar levels.

Chapter 10: Eating Out and Traveling with Diabetes

Choosing Restaurants Wisely

Traveling can present unique challenges for individuals with diabetes, especially when it comes to dining out at restaurants. Here are some tips for choosing restaurants wisely while traveling:

Research Ahead

Before your trip, research restaurants in the area where you'll be staying. Look for eateries that offer healthy and diabetic-friendly options on their menu. Many restaurants now provide their menus online, making it easier to plan ahead.

Look for Healthy Options

When choosing a restaurant, opt for establishments that offer a variety of healthy options such as grilled or baked lean proteins, steamed or roasted vegetables, whole grains, and salads with lean protein toppings. Avoid restaurants known for their deep-fried or heavily processed dishes.

Consider Portion Sizes

Pay attention to portion sizes when dining out. Many restaurants serve oversized portions, which can contribute to overeating and blood sugar spikes. Consider sharing an entree with a travel companion or ask for a half-portion if available.

Ask Questions

Don't hesitate to ask your server questions about how dishes are prepared. Inquire about ingredients, cooking methods, and any modifications that can be made to accommodate your dietary needs. Most restaurants are willing to accommodate special requests.

Customize Your Order

Don't be afraid to customize your order to suit your dietary preferences and needs. Ask for dressings and sauces on the side, request steamed vegetables instead of fried, and opt for whole grain or vegetable-based substitutions when possible.

Beware of Hidden Sugars

Be mindful of hidden sugars in restaurant dishes, especially in sauces, dressings, and marinades. Ask for sauces and dressings to be served on the side so you can control the amount you use, or request sugar-free alternatives.

Practice Portion Control

If you're dining at a buffet or all-you-can-eat restaurant, practice portion control by filling your plate with mostly vegetables, lean proteins, and whole grains. Limit your intake of high-carb and high-calorie dishes, and avoid going back for seconds.

Stay Hydrated

Remember to stay hydrated while dining out by drinking water or unsweetened beverages. Limit your intake of sugary drinks like soda, sweet tea, and cocktails, which can contribute to blood sugar spikes.

By choosing restaurants wisely and making informed choices while dining out, you can enjoy delicious meals while managing your diabetes effectively during your travels. Remember to listen to your body and prioritize your health and well-being.

Navigating the Menu

When traveling with diabetes, navigating restaurant menus can seem daunting. Here are some tips to help you make healthy choices while dining out:

Scan the Menu Carefully

Take your time to review the menu thoroughly. Look for keywords such as "grilled," "baked," "steamed," and "fresh" which often indicate healthier cooking methods and options.

Focus on Protein and Vegetables

Build your meal around lean protein sources such as grilled chicken, fish, tofu, or lean cuts of beef or pork. Pair your protein with a generous serving of vegetables, which are low in calories and high in fiber, vitamins, and minerals.

Watch Out for Hidden Carbs

Be cautious of dishes that are heavy on refined carbohydrates such as white bread, pasta, rice, and potatoes. Instead, opt for whole grain or vegetable-based alternatives when available to help stabilize blood sugar levels.

Ask for Modifications

Don't hesitate to ask your server for modifications to suit your dietary needs. Request steamed or sautéed vegetables instead of fried, ask for sauces and dressings on the side, and opt for whole grain or lettuce wraps instead of bread or tortillas.

Choose Healthy Cooking Methods

Look for dishes that are prepared using healthier cooking methods such as grilling, baking, steaming, or broiling. Avoid dishes that are deep-fried, breaded, or coated in heavy sauces, which can add unnecessary calories and fat.

Portion Control

Be mindful of portion sizes, especially when dining out at restaurants known for their large servings. Consider sharing an entree with a travel companion or ask for a half-portion if available to avoid overeating and blood sugar spikes.

Be Wary of Salad Traps

While salads can be a healthy option, they can also be loaded with hidden sugars, fats, and calories in the form of creamy dressings, cheese, croutons, and candied nuts. Opt for salads with lean protein toppings and dressing on the side, or create your own salad by choosing fresh vegetables and a lean protein source.

Stay Hydrated

Don't forget to stay hydrated by drinking water or unsweetened beverages with your meal. Limit your intake of sugary drinks like soda, sweet tea, and alcoholic beverages, which can contribute to blood sugar spikes.

By navigating the menu with these tips in mind, you can make informed choices that support your diabetes management goals while enjoying delicious meals during your travels. Remember to listen to your body and prioritize your health and well-being.

Travel Tips for Diabetics

Traveling with diabetes requires some extra planning and preparation to ensure a smooth and enjoyable trip. Here are some helpful tips to help you manage your diabetes while traveling:

Pack Supplies Wisely

Make sure to pack all necessary diabetes supplies, including blood glucose monitoring devices, test strips, insulin or oral medications, syringes or insulin pens, lancets, glucose tablets or gel, and any other medications or supplies you may need. Pack extra supplies in case of emergencies or unexpected delays.

Carry Snacks

Always carry a supply of healthy snacks with you, such as nuts, seeds, whole grain crackers, fresh fruit, or low-fat cheese. Having snacks on hand can help prevent low blood sugar levels (hypoglycemia) and provide a quick source of energy while traveling.

Stay Hydrated

Drink plenty of water throughout your journey to stay hydrated, especially if you're flying or spending time in a dry environment. Avoid sugary drinks and alcoholic beverages, which can contribute to dehydration and blood sugar fluctuations.

Plan Meals and Snacks

Research restaurants and grocery stores at your destination ahead of time to ensure access to healthy food options. Consider packing some meals and snacks for travel days to avoid relying on airport or roadside options that may be high in sugar and unhealthy fats.

Keep Medications Handy

Keep your medications and supplies easily accessible during your travels. Store insulin and other medications in a travel cooler or insulated bag to protect them from extreme temperatures. Carry a letter from your healthcare provider explaining your condition and the need for carrying medications and supplies, especially when traveling internationally.

Monitor Blood Sugar Levels

Regularly monitor your blood sugar levels throughout your journey, especially during long flights or car rides. Changes in routine, time zone differences, and physical activity levels can all affect blood sugar levels, so be vigilant and adjust your insulin or medication doses as needed.

Stay Active

Incorporate physical activity into your travel itinerary whenever possible. Take short walks during layovers, stretch your legs during long flights, and explore your destination on foot whenever feasible. Regular exercise can help regulate blood sugar levels and improve overall well-being.

Stay Informed

Familiarize yourself with local healthcare facilities and emergency services at your destination. Carry a diabetes ID card or wear a medical alert bracelet or necklace to alert others of your condition in case of an emergency.

Manage Stress

Traveling can be stressful, which can affect blood sugar levels. Practice stress-reducing techniques such as deep breathing, meditation, or yoga to help keep stress levels in check during your journey.

By following these travel tips for diabetes, you can enjoy a safe and enjoyable trip while effectively managing your diabetes away from home. Remember to plan ahead, stay prepared, and prioritize your health and well-being throughout your travels.

Managing Diabetes on Vacation

Vacations are a time to relax, unwind, and explore new destinations, but managing diabetes while on vacation requires some extra planning and preparation. Here are some tips to help you enjoy a stress-free vacation while effectively managing your diabetes:

Plan Ahead

Before your trip, take the time to plan and prepare for managing your diabetes while on vacation. Research your destination to familiarize yourself with local healthcare facilities, pharmacies, and emergency services. Pack all necessary diabetes supplies, medications, and snacks to last the duration of your trip.

Stick to Your Routine

While it's tempting to let loose and indulge on vacation, try to stick to your regular diabetes management routine as much as possible. Maintain consistent meal times, monitor your blood sugar levels regularly, and take your medications or insulin doses as prescribed by your healthcare provider.

Choose Accommodations Wisely

When booking accommodations, consider factors such as access to kitchen facilities, refrigerator availability for storing insulin, and proximity to grocery stores or restaurants with diabetic-friendly options. Renting a vacation home or apartment with a kitchen can provide more flexibility in meal planning and preparation.

Stay Active

Incorporate physical activity into your vacation itinerary to help regulate blood sugar levels and maintain overall health. Take advantage of opportunities for sightseeing on foot, swimming, hiking, or participating in local recreational activities. Pack comfortable walking shoes and workout attire to stay active while exploring your destination.

Stay Hydrated

Drink plenty of water throughout your vacation to stay hydrated, especially if you're spending time outdoors in warm weather or engaging in physical activities. Avoid sugary drinks and alcoholic beverages, which can contribute to dehydration and blood sugar fluctuations.

Plan Meals and Snacks

Research restaurants and dining options at your destination ahead of time to ensure access to healthy food choices. Look for restaurants that offer diabetic-friendly options or customizable menu items. Consider packing some healthy snacks for travel days and day trips to avoid relying on high-carb or unhealthy options.

Monitor Blood Sugar Levels

Regularly monitor your blood sugar levels throughout your vacation, especially if you're changing time zones or engaging in different activities than usual. Keep a log of your blood sugar readings and any symptoms you experience to track patterns and make adjustments as needed.

Communicate with Travel Companions

If you're traveling with friends or family, communicate with them about your diabetes management needs and how they can support you during your vacation. Ensure they know how to recognize and respond to signs of low blood sugar (hypoglycemia) and have access to your emergency contact information.

Be Prepared for Emergencies

Carry a diabetes ID card, medical alert bracelet or necklace, and a letter from your healthcare provider explaining your condition and the need for carrying medications and supplies. Familiarize yourself with local emergency services and healthcare facilities at your destination in case of unexpected medical issues.

Relax and Enjoy

Most importantly, relax and enjoy your vacation! Don't let diabetes hold you back from experiencing new adventures and making lasting memories. With careful planning, preparation, and self-care, you can enjoy a safe and fulfilling vacation while effectively managing your diabetes.

By following these tips for managing diabetes on vacation, you can enjoy a stress-free and memorable getaway while prioritizing your health and well-being. Remember to plan ahead, stay prepared, and listen to your body throughout your travels.

Chapter 11: Alcohol and Diabetes

Effects of Alcohol on Blood Sugar

Alcohol consumption can have a significant impact on blood sugar levels, especially for individuals with diabetes. Understanding how alcohol affects blood sugar is essential for managing diabetes effectively. Here are some key points to consider:

Immediate Effect on Blood Sugar

Alcohol is quickly absorbed into the bloodstream, leading to a rapid increase in blood alcohol concentration (BAC). Initially, alcohol may cause blood sugar levels to rise, particularly if consumed on an empty stomach or in large quantities.

Delayed Hypoglycemia

Despite the initial rise in blood sugar, alcohol can also lead to delayed hypoglycemia, or low blood sugar levels, several hours after consumption. This is because alcohol impairs the liver's ability to produce glucose, which can lead to a drop in blood sugar levels.

Risk of Hypoglycemia

For individuals taking insulin or certain diabetes medications, the risk of hypoglycemia is heightened when consuming alcohol. This is especially true if alcohol is consumed without food or in conjunction with medications that lower blood sugar levels.

Caloric Content

Alcoholic beverages are often high in calories but low in nutrients, which can contribute to weight gain and poor blood sugar control if consumed in excess. It's important to be mindful of the calorie content of alcoholic drinks and choose lower-calorie options whenever possible.

Interference with Diabetes Medications

Alcohol can interact with certain diabetes medications, including insulin and oral hypoglycemic agents, leading to unpredictable changes in blood sugar levels. It's important to consult with a healthcare provider or pharmacist about potential interactions before consuming alcohol.

Hydration Status

Alcohol is a diuretic, meaning it increases urine production and can lead to dehydration if not consumed in moderation. Dehydration can exacerbate the symptoms of high blood sugar and increase the risk of hypoglycemia.

Impact on Judgment

Alcohol can impair judgment and decision-making, which may lead to poor food choices or forgetting to monitor blood sugar levels. It's important to drink alcohol responsibly and monitor blood sugar levels closely, especially when away from home or in social settings.

Moderation is Key

While moderate alcohol consumption may be safe for some individuals with diabetes, excessive or binge drinking can have serious health consequences and should be avoided. The American Diabetes Association recommends limiting alcohol intake to one drink per day for women and up to two drinks per day for men, with a drink defined as 12 ounces of beer, 5 ounces of wine, or 1.5 ounces of distilled spirits.

By understanding the effects of alcohol on blood sugar and practicing moderation, individuals with diabetes can enjoy alcoholic beverages responsibly while minimizing the risk of adverse effects on blood sugar control and overall health. It's important to consult with a healthcare provider or diabetes educator for personalized guidance on alcohol consumption and diabetes management.

Safe Drinking Guidelines

For individuals with diabetes, consuming alcohol can pose unique challenges and risks. However, with careful planning and moderation, it is possible to enjoy alcoholic beverages responsibly while managing diabetes effectively. Here are some safe drinking guidelines to keep in mind:

Consult with Healthcare Provider

Before consuming alcohol, especially if you have diabetes, it's important to consult with your healthcare provider or diabetes educator. They can provide personalized guidance based on your individual health status, medications, and blood sugar control goals.

Know Your Limits

Understand your personal tolerance for alcohol and know your limits. The American Diabetes Association recommends limiting alcohol intake to one drink per day for women and up to two drinks per day for men, with a drink defined as 12 ounces of beer, 5 ounces of wine, or 1.5 ounces of distilled spirits.

Monitor Blood Sugar Levels

Before, during, and after consuming alcohol, monitor your blood sugar levels closely. Alcohol can cause fluctuations in blood sugar levels, so it's essential to check your levels regularly and be prepared to take action if necessary.

Never Drink on an Empty Stomach

Consuming alcohol on an empty stomach can lead to rapid spikes or drops in blood sugar levels. Always eat a balanced meal or snack containing carbohydrates, protein, and healthy fats before drinking alcohol to help stabilize blood sugar levels.

Stay Hydrated

Alternate alcoholic beverages with water or other non-alcoholic, sugar-free drinks to stay hydrated and prevent dehydration. Alcohol is a diuretic and can lead to increased urine output, which can contribute to dehydration if not balanced with adequate fluid intake.

Avoid Sugary Mixers

Choose alcoholic beverages that are low in sugar and calories, and avoid sugary mixers such as regular soda, fruit juice, or flavored syrups. Opt for sugar-free mixers like club soda, diet tonic water, or sparkling water instead.

Beware of Hidden Calories

Alcoholic beverages can be high in calories and may contribute to weight gain if consumed in excess. Be mindful of portion sizes and choose lower-calorie options whenever possible. Light beer, dry wine, and distilled spirits mixed with calorie-free mixers are generally lower in calories than sweet cocktails or heavy beers.

Don't Drink and Drive

Never drink and drive, especially if you have diabetes. Alcohol can impair judgment, coordination, and reaction time, making it dangerous to operate a vehicle. Arrange for a designated driver, use public transportation, or call a taxi or rideshare service if you've been drinking.

Be Prepared for Emergencies

Carry diabetes supplies, such as glucose tablets or gel, with you at all times when drinking alcohol. Know the signs and symptoms of low blood sugar (hypoglycemia) and how to treat it promptly if it occurs.

Listen to Your Body

Pay attention to how alcohol affects your body and blood sugar levels. If you experience any adverse effects or symptoms, such as dizziness, nausea, confusion, or changes in vision, stop drinking and seek medical attention if necessary.

By following these safe drinking guidelines, individuals with diabetes can enjoy alcoholic beverages responsibly while minimizing the risk of adverse effects on blood sugar control and overall health. Remember that moderation is key, and always prioritize your health and well-being when consuming alcohol.

Alcohol and Hypoglycemia

Hypoglycemia, or low blood sugar levels, is a concern for individuals with diabetes, especially when consuming alcohol. Alcohol can affect blood sugar levels in various ways, increasing the risk of hypoglycemia if not managed properly. Here's how alcohol can contribute to hypoglycemia and tips for preventing and managing it:

Delayed Hypoglycemia

While alcohol initially raises blood sugar levels by inhibiting the liver's release of glucose, it can lead to delayed hypoglycemia several hours after consumption. This is because alcohol impairs the liver's ability to produce glucose, which is needed to maintain blood sugar levels, leading to a drop in blood sugar levels over time.

Masking Symptoms

Alcohol can mask the symptoms of hypoglycemia, making it more difficult to recognize and treat low blood sugar levels. Symptoms of hypoglycemia, such as dizziness, confusion, sweating, and shakiness, may be mistaken for the effects of alcohol intoxication, leading to delayed or inadequate treatment.

Increased Sensitivity to Insulin

Alcohol can increase insulin sensitivity, especially in individuals with type 1 diabetes who take insulin injections. This means that the insulin you've already taken may have a stronger effect when combined with alcohol, leading to a greater risk of hypoglycemia.

Dehydration

Alcohol is a diuretic, meaning it increases urine production and can lead to dehydration if not balanced with adequate fluid intake. Dehydration can exacerbate the symptoms of hypoglycemia and increase the risk of complications.

Preventing Hypoglycemia

To prevent hypoglycemia when drinking alcohol, it's essential to plan ahead and take precautions. Eat a balanced meal or snack containing carbohydrates, protein, and healthy fats before drinking alcohol to help stabilize blood sugar levels. Monitor your blood sugar levels closely before, during, and after drinking alcohol, and be prepared to treat hypoglycemia promptly if it occurs.

Carry Glucose

Always carry a source of fast-acting glucose, such as glucose tablets, gel, or hard candy, with you when drinking alcohol. If you experience symptoms of hypoglycemia, such as dizziness, confusion, or sweating, consume a serving of glucose to raise your blood sugar levels quickly.

Avoid Excessive Drinking

Excessive alcohol consumption can increase the risk of hypoglycemia and other complications, especially for individuals with diabetes. Stick to moderate drinking guidelines and avoid binge drinking or heavy alcohol consumption.

Communicate with Others

If you're drinking alcohol with friends or family, communicate with them about your diabetes and the signs and symptoms of hypoglycemia. Make sure they know how to recognize and respond to low blood sugar levels and have access to your emergency contact information.

By understanding the relationship between alcohol and hypoglycemia and taking appropriate precautions, individuals with diabetes can enjoy alcoholic beverages responsibly while minimizing the risk of low blood sugar levels and related complications. Remember to monitor your blood sugar levels closely, carry glucose with you at all times, and prioritize your health and well-being when consuming alcohol.

Choosing Diabetic-Friendly Drinks

When it comes to enjoying alcoholic beverages with diabetes, making smart choices is key to managing blood sugar levels effectively. Here are some tips for choosing diabetic-friendly drinks:

Opt for Low-Carb Options

Choose alcoholic beverages that are low in carbohydrates to help minimize the impact on blood sugar levels. Examples of low-carb options include:

- Light beer or non-alcoholic beer

- Dry wines such as Chardonnay, Pinot Grigio, or Sauvignon Blanc

- Distilled spirits such as vodka, gin, rum, whiskey, or tequila, served straight or with calorie-free mixers like club soda or diet tonic water

Avoid Sugary Mixers

Sugary mixers such as regular soda, fruit juice, tonic water, and sweetened syrups can significantly increase the carbohydrate content of your drink and lead to blood sugar spikes. Instead, choose sugar-free mixers or enjoy your alcoholic beverages neat or on the rocks.

Watch Portion Sizes

Be mindful of portion sizes when drinking alcoholic beverages, as larger servings can contain more carbohydrates and calories. Stick to standard serving sizes and avoid oversized drinks or heavy pours.

Monitor Blood Sugar Levels

Regularly monitor your blood sugar levels before, during, and after drinking alcoholic beverages to track how they affect your body. Keep a log of your blood sugar readings and any symptoms you experience to identify patterns and make adjustments as needed.

Stay Hydrated

Alcohol is a diuretic, meaning it increases urine production and can lead to dehydration if not balanced with adequate fluid intake. Drink plenty of water alongside alcoholic beverages to stay hydrated and help prevent dehydration.

Avoid Artificial Sweeteners

Some sugar-free mixers and diet sodas contain artificial sweeteners, which may affect blood sugar levels and insulin sensitivity in some individuals. If you're sensitive to artificial sweeteners, choose mixers that are naturally sugar-free, such as club soda or sparkling water.

Limit Cocktails and Frozen Drinks

Cocktails and frozen drinks often contain added sugars, syrups, and high-calorie mixers, making them less suitable for individuals with diabetes. Limit your intake of these high-calorie, high-carb options and opt for lighter alternatives instead.

Practice Moderation

Moderation is key when it comes to drinking alcoholic beverages with diabetes. Stick to recommended guidelines for moderate alcohol consumption, which include up to one drink per day for women and up to two drinks per day for men.

By choosing diabetic-friendly drinks and practicing moderation, individuals with diabetes can enjoy alcoholic beverages responsibly while minimizing the impact on blood sugar levels and overall health. Remember to monitor blood sugar levels closely, stay hydrated, and prioritize your well-being when enjoying alcoholic beverages.

Chapter 12: Diabetes and Pregnancy

Managing Diabetes During Pregnancy

Pregnancy is an exciting and joyful time, but it can also present unique challenges for women with diabetes. Proper management of diabetes during pregnancy is essential to ensure the health and well-being of both the mother and the baby. Here are some key strategies for managing diabetes during pregnancy:

Preconception Planning

If you have diabetes and are planning to conceive, it's important to work closely with your healthcare provider to optimize your blood sugar control before becoming pregnant. Preconception planning can help reduce the risk of complications during pregnancy and improve outcomes for both mother and baby.

Regular Prenatal Care

Attend regular prenatal appointments with your healthcare provider to monitor your blood sugar levels, assess fetal growth and development, and address any concerns or complications that may arise. Prenatal care is essential for managing diabetes during pregnancy and ensuring a healthy pregnancy and delivery.

Blood Sugar Monitoring

Monitor your blood sugar levels closely throughout pregnancy, as hormonal changes and increased insulin resistance can affect blood sugar control. Your healthcare provider may recommend more frequent blood sugar monitoring, including fasting, pre-meal, and post-meal readings, to ensure optimal blood sugar control.

Healthy Eating

Follow a balanced and nutritious diet during pregnancy, focusing on whole foods, lean proteins, fruits, vegetables, and whole grains. Work with a registered dietitian or certified diabetes educator to develop a personalized meal plan that meets your nutritional needs and helps regulate blood sugar levels.

Physical Activity

Stay physically active during pregnancy, as regular exercise can help improve blood sugar control, reduce insulin resistance, and promote overall health and well-being. Aim for at least 30 minutes of moderate-intensity exercise most days of the week, as recommended by your healthcare provider.

Medication Management

If you take insulin or oral medications to manage diabetes, continue taking your prescribed medications as directed by your healthcare provider. Your medication regimen may need to be adjusted during pregnancy to maintain optimal blood sugar control.

Gestational Diabetes Screening

Women with diabetes are at increased risk of developing gestational diabetes, a form of diabetes that occurs during pregnancy. Your healthcare provider will likely screen you for gestational diabetes between 24 and 28 weeks of pregnancy using an oral glucose tolerance test (OGTT).

Complications Monitoring

Be aware of potential complications associated with diabetes during pregnancy, including preeclampsia, preterm labor, macrosomia (large baby), and neonatal hypoglycemia. Attend all recommended prenatal appointments and contact your healthcare provider immediately if you experience any symptoms or concerns.

Emotional Support

Pregnancy can be an emotional time, especially for women with diabetes who may have concerns about their health and the health of their baby. Seek emotional support from loved ones, support groups, or mental health professionals to help cope with the challenges of managing diabetes during pregnancy.

Postpartum Care

After delivery, continue to monitor your blood sugar levels closely and attend postpartum follow-up appointments with your healthcare provider. Breastfeeding can help regulate blood sugar levels in the postpartum period, but adjustments to medication may be necessary.

By following these strategies for managing diabetes during pregnancy and working closely with your healthcare provider, you can enjoy a healthy pregnancy and give your baby the best possible start in life. Remember that proper blood sugar control is essential for the health and well-being of both you and your baby, and don't hesitate to reach out for support when needed.

Nutrition for Pregnant Diabetics

Maintaining a healthy diet is crucial for pregnant women with diabetes to ensure optimal blood sugar control and support the growth and development of the baby. Here are some key principles of nutrition for pregnant women with diabetes:

Balanced Meals

Aim to eat balanced meals that include a combination of carbohydrates, protein, and healthy fats. Spread your carbohydrate intake evenly throughout the day to help regulate blood sugar levels and avoid large fluctuations.

Choose Complex Carbohydrates

Focus on consuming complex carbohydrates that are high in fiber and low on the glycemic index, such as whole grains, legumes, fruits, and vegetables. These carbohydrates are digested more slowly, leading to gradual increases in blood sugar levels.

Monitor Portion Sizes

Be mindful of portion sizes to avoid overeating and blood sugar spikes. Use measuring cups, food scales, or visual cues to help you portion out your meals and snacks appropriately.

Include Lean Protein

Incorporate lean sources of protein into your meals and snacks to help stabilize blood sugar levels and promote satiety. Good sources of protein include poultry, fish, lean cuts of meat, tofu, eggs, dairy products, and plant-based protein sources like beans and lentils.

Healthy Fats

Include sources of healthy fats in your diet, such as avocados, nuts, seeds, olive oil, and fatty fish like salmon and sardines. Healthy fats help provide essential nutrients and support the baby's brain and eye development.

Limit Saturated and Trans Fats

Minimize your intake of saturated and trans fats, which can increase the risk of heart disease and other health complications. Choose lean cuts of meat, low-fat dairy products, and healthier cooking methods like baking, grilling, or steaming.

Stay Hydrated

Drink plenty of water throughout the day to stay hydrated and support overall health and well-being. Limit your intake of sugary beverages and opt for water, herbal tea, or sparkling water instead.

Meal Timing

Space out your meals and snacks evenly throughout the day to help regulate blood sugar levels and prevent large fluctuations. Aim to eat every 3-4 hours to maintain steady energy levels and avoid dips in blood sugar.

Monitor Blood Sugar Levels

Regularly monitor your blood sugar levels before and after meals, as well as fasting and bedtime readings. Keep a log of your blood sugar readings and any symptoms you experience to track patterns and make adjustments to your diet and medication regimen as needed.

Seek Guidance

Work with a registered dietitian or certified diabetes educator who specializes in prenatal nutrition to develop a personalized meal plan that meets your nutritional needs and supports optimal blood sugar control during pregnancy.

By following these principles of nutrition for pregnant women with diabetes, you can support a healthy pregnancy, ensure optimal blood sugar control, and give your baby the best possible start in life. Remember to prioritize your health and well-being throughout your pregnancy journey and seek support from healthcare professionals as needed.

Gestational Diabetes

Gestational diabetes mellitus (GDM) is a form of diabetes that develops during pregnancy, usually in the second or third trimester. It is characterized by high blood sugar levels that can pose risks to both the mother and the baby if not properly managed. Here's what you need to know about gestational diabetes:

Risk Factors

Women who are overweight or obese, have a family history of diabetes, or have previously had gestational diabetes are at increased risk of developing GDM. Other risk factors include being older than age 25, having polycystic ovary syndrome (PCOS), and certain ethnic backgrounds, such as Hispanic, African American, Native American, or Asian.

Screening

Most pregnant women are screened for gestational diabetes between 24 and 28 weeks of pregnancy using an oral glucose tolerance test (OGTT). This test involves drinking a sugary beverage and then having blood sugar levels tested at specific intervals to determine how well the body metabolizes glucose.

Complications

Untreated or poorly controlled gestational diabetes can lead to various complications for both the mother and the baby. These may include macrosomia (large baby), birth trauma, preterm birth, preeclampsia (high blood pressure during pregnancy), cesarean delivery, and an increased risk of developing type 2 diabetes later in life for both mother and child.

Management

The primary goal of managing gestational diabetes is to keep blood sugar levels within target ranges to minimize the risk of complications. This often involves making dietary and lifestyle changes, monitoring blood sugar levels regularly, and, in some cases, taking insulin or oral medications to help control blood sugar levels.

Nutrition

Nutrition plays a crucial role in managing gestational diabetes. Pregnant women with GDM are typically advised to follow a balanced diet that includes a variety of nutrient-dense foods, with a focus on complex carbohydrates, lean proteins, healthy fats, and plenty of fruits and vegetables. Portion control, spacing out meals and snacks, and avoiding sugary and processed foods are also important.

Physical Activity

Regular physical activity can help improve blood sugar control and reduce the risk of complications associated with gestational diabetes. Pregnant women with GDM are encouraged to engage in moderate-intensity exercise most days of the week, as recommended by their healthcare provider.

Monitoring

Pregnant women with gestational diabetes will need to monitor their blood sugar levels regularly, typically several times a day. This may involve testing fasting blood sugar levels in the morning, as well as postprandial (after meals) blood sugar levels to ensure they stay within target ranges.

Medical Management

In some cases, dietary and lifestyle changes may not be enough to control blood sugar levels, and medication may be necessary. Insulin is the most common medication used to treat gestational diabetes, although oral medications may also be prescribed in some cases.

Follow-Up Care

After delivery, blood sugar levels usually return to normal, but women who have had gestational diabetes are at increased risk of developing type 2 diabetes later in life. It's important to attend postpartum follow-up appointments and continue monitoring blood sugar levels regularly to detect any signs of diabetes early on.

By understanding the risk factors, complications, and management strategies associated with gestational diabetes, women can take proactive steps to ensure a healthy pregnancy and reduce the risk of complications for both themselves and their babies. Working closely with healthcare providers and following recommended guidelines for nutrition, physical activity, and blood sugar monitoring can help women with gestational diabetes manage their condition effectively and enjoy a healthy pregnancy.

Postpartum Care for Diabetic Mothers

The postpartum period, or the time following childbirth, is a crucial phase for diabetic mothers to focus on their health and well-being. Proper postpartum care is essential for managing diabetes, promoting recovery, and supporting overall health during this transitional period. Here are some key aspects of postpartum care for diabetic mothers:

Blood Sugar Monitoring

It's important to continue monitoring blood sugar levels regularly in the postpartum period, as hormonal changes and fluctuations can affect blood sugar control. Your healthcare provider may recommend checking blood sugar levels more frequently during this time, especially if you had gestational diabetes or preexisting diabetes.

Nutrition and Hydration

Maintain a balanced diet that supports postpartum recovery and blood sugar control. Focus on nutrient-dense foods such as fruits, vegetables, whole grains, lean proteins, and healthy fats. Stay hydrated by drinking plenty of water throughout the day, especially if breastfeeding.

Physical Activity

Gradually reintroduce physical activity into your routine as your body heals from childbirth. Consult with your healthcare provider before starting any exercise regimen and aim for regular, moderate-intensity activity that promotes cardiovascular health and helps manage blood sugar levels.

Medication Management

If you were taking insulin or oral medications to manage diabetes during pregnancy, your medication regimen may need to be adjusted in the postpartum period. Work closely with your healthcare provider to determine the appropriate dosage and timing of medications to maintain optimal blood sugar control.

Breastfeeding Support

If you choose to breastfeed, it's important to monitor blood sugar levels closely, as breastfeeding can affect insulin sensitivity and blood sugar levels. Consult with a lactation consultant or healthcare provider for guidance on breastfeeding and managing diabetes while nursing.

Emotional Well-Being

The postpartum period can be emotionally challenging for many mothers, including those with diabetes. Be proactive about prioritizing self-care, seeking support from loved ones, and reaching out to healthcare providers or mental health professionals if you experience feelings of depression, anxiety, or stress.

Follow-Up Care

Attend all postpartum follow-up appointments with your healthcare provider to monitor your recovery, assess blood sugar control, and address any concerns or complications that may arise. Be proactive about discussing your diabetes management plan and any changes in your health status since giving birth.

Family Planning

If you're considering future pregnancies, discuss family planning options and strategies for managing diabetes during pregnancy with your healthcare provider. Planning ahead can help optimize your health and minimize risks for future pregnancies.

By prioritizing postpartum care and taking proactive steps to manage diabetes effectively, diabetic mothers can support their own health and well-being while caring for their newborns. Remember to reach out for support from healthcare providers, loved ones, and community resources as needed during this transitional period.

Chapter 13: Diabetes in Children and Adolescents

Type 1 Diabetes in Kids

Diabetes is a chronic condition that affects people of all ages, including children and adolescents. Managing diabetes in kids requires careful attention to diet, physical activity, medication, and overall health. The two main types of diabetes that can occur in children i.e type 1 diabetes and type 2 diabetes. Type 2 diabetes, once considered an adult-onset condition, is becoming increasingly common in children and adolescents, particularly those who are overweight or obese.

Symptoms

The symptoms of diabetes in children are similar to those in adults and may include increased thirst, frequent urination, unexplained weight loss, fatigue, blurred vision, and slow wound healing. If you notice any of these symptoms in your child, it's important to seek medical attention promptly for evaluation and diagnosis.

Diagnosis

Diagnosing diabetes in children typically involves blood tests to measure blood sugar levels. For type 1 diabetes, additional tests such as the presence of autoantibodies may be performed to confirm the diagnosis. For type 2 diabetes, other risk factors such as family history, obesity, and physical inactivity may also be considered.

Treatment

The primary goals of treating diabetes in children are to maintain blood sugar levels within target ranges, prevent complications, and support overall health and well-being. Treatment may involve a combination of insulin therapy, oral medications (for type 2 diabetes), dietary modifications, regular physical activity, and close monitoring of blood sugar levels.

Dietary Management

A healthy diet plays a crucial role in managing diabetes in children. Encourage your child to eat a balanced diet that includes a variety of nutrient-dense foods, with an emphasis on fruits, vegetables, whole grains, lean proteins, and healthy fats. Limit sugary and processed foods, and encourage portion control to help regulate blood sugar levels.

Physical Activity

Regular physical activity is important for children with diabetes to help improve insulin sensitivity, control weight, and promote overall health. Encourage your child to engage in age-appropriate activities they enjoy, such as sports, swimming, biking, or dancing, and aim for at least 60 minutes of moderate to vigorous activity most days of the week.

Medication Management

Children with type 1 diabetes require insulin therapy to replace the insulin their bodies no longer produce. Insulin may be administered via injections or an insulin pump, depending on individual needs and preferences. Children with type 2 diabetes may also require oral medications or, in some cases, insulin therapy to help manage blood sugar levels.

Emotional Support

Living with diabetes can be challenging for children and their families, both physically and emotionally. Provide emotional support and encouragement to your child, and involve them in their diabetes management to the extent possible. Connect with support groups, healthcare providers, and mental health professionals as needed to address any concerns or difficulties.

Education and Empowerment

Educate your child about diabetes and empower them to take an active role in managing their condition. Teach them how to check their blood sugar levels, administer insulin (if applicable), recognize and respond to symptoms of high or low blood sugar, and make healthy lifestyle choices.

Regular Monitoring and Follow-Up

Schedule regular check-ups with your child's healthcare provider to monitor blood sugar levels, assess overall health, and adjust treatment as needed. Stay informed about advances in diabetes management and treatment options, and advocate for your child's health and well-being.

By taking a proactive approach to managing diabetes in children and adolescents, parents and caregivers can help their children lead healthy, active lives while effectively managing their condition. Remember to prioritize open communication, education, and support to empower your child to thrive despite diabetes.

Nutrition for Diabetic Kids

Proper nutrition plays a vital role in managing diabetes in children and adolescents. A healthy diet helps regulate blood sugar levels, supports growth and development, and reduces the risk of complications associated with diabetes. Here are some key principles of nutrition for kids with diabetes:

Balanced Meals

Encourage your child to eat balanced meals that include a variety of nutrient-dense foods from all food groups. Aim for a combination of carbohydrates, protein, and healthy fats at each meal to help stabilize blood sugar levels and provide sustained energy.

Carbohydrate Counting

Carbohydrates have the most significant impact on blood sugar levels, so it's essential to monitor carbohydrate intake carefully. Teach your child how to count carbohydrates and adjust insulin doses accordingly, especially if they use insulin therapy to manage diabetes.

Choose Healthy Carbohydrates

Focus on incorporating healthy carbohydrates into your child's diet, such as whole grains, fruits, vegetables, legumes, and low-fat dairy products. These foods are rich in fiber, vitamins, and minerals and are digested more slowly, leading to gradual increases in blood sugar levels.

Portion Control

Pay attention to portion sizes to avoid overeating and blood sugar spikes. Use measuring cups, food scales, or visual cues to help your child portion out their meals and snacks appropriately. Avoid super-sized portions and encourage your child to listen to their body's hunger and fullness cues.

Limit Sugary and Processed Foods

Minimize your child's intake of sugary and processed foods, including sweets, candies, sugary beverages, and processed snacks. These foods can cause rapid spikes in blood sugar levels and contribute to weight gain and other health complications.

Encourage Regular Meals and Snacks

Encourage your child to eat regular meals and snacks throughout the day to help maintain stable blood sugar levels. Skipping meals or going too long without eating can lead to fluctuations in blood sugar levels and may increase the risk of hypoglycemia (low blood sugar).

Healthy Snack Options

Provide your child with a variety of healthy snack options that are low in sugar and high in protein, fiber, and healthy fats. Examples include fresh fruit with nut butter, Greek yogurt with berries, whole grain crackers with cheese, or vegetable sticks with hummus.

Stay Hydrated

Make sure your child stays hydrated by drinking plenty of water throughout the day. Water is the best choice for hydration, but low-calorie beverages such as herbal tea or infused water can also be refreshing options.

Model Healthy Eating Habits

Set a positive example for your child by modeling healthy eating habits and making nutritious food choices yourself. Involve your child in meal planning, grocery shopping, and cooking to help them develop lifelong healthy eating habits.

Seek Support

Work with a registered dietitian or certified diabetes educator who specializes in pediatric nutrition to develop a personalized meal plan that meets your child's nutritional needs and supports optimal blood sugar control. Connect with support groups, healthcare providers, and other families affected by diabetes for additional guidance and support.

By focusing on nutritious, balanced meals, monitoring carbohydrate intake, and promoting healthy eating habits, parents and caregivers can help children and adolescents with diabetes manage their condition effectively and enjoy a happy, healthy childhood. Remember that every child is unique, so it's essential to tailor nutrition recommendations to meet your child's individual needs and preferences.

Managing Diabetes at School

Managing diabetes at school is crucial for children and adolescents with diabetes to ensure their safety, well-being, and academic success. Effective communication, education, and collaboration among parents, school staff, and healthcare providers are essential for creating a supportive environment for students with diabetes. Here are some key strategies for managing diabetes at school:

Develop a Diabetes Management Plan

Work with your child's healthcare provider to develop a comprehensive diabetes management plan that outlines their specific needs, medication regimen, blood sugar monitoring schedule, dietary considerations, emergency procedures, and other relevant information. Share this plan with school staff, including teachers, administrators, school nurses, and other personnel who may interact with your child during the school day.

Educate School Staff

Provide education and training to school staff about diabetes, its management, and how to recognize and respond to hypo- and hyperglycemia. Ensure that key personnel, such as teachers, coaches, cafeteria staff, bus drivers, and school nurses, are familiar with your child's diabetes management plan and know how to administer insulin, check blood sugar levels, and respond to emergency situations.

Promote Self-Care Skills

Teach your child age-appropriate self-care skills to manage their diabetes independently at school. This may include checking blood sugar levels, administering insulin injections or using an insulin pump, counting carbohydrates, recognizing symptoms of hypo- and hyperglycemia, and knowing when and how to seek help from school staff.

Provide Emergency Supplies

Ensure that your child has access to emergency supplies and medications at school, including glucose tablets or gel, fast-acting carbohydrates, a blood glucose meter, insulin, glucagon emergency kits, and contact information for parents or guardians and healthcare providers. Keep these supplies in a designated location that is easily accessible to your child and school staff in case of an emergency.

Accommodate Mealtime Needs

Work with school staff to accommodate your child's mealtime needs, including providing access to nutritious meals and snacks, allowing time for blood sugar checks and insulin administration before meals, and ensuring that your child can eat safely in the classroom, cafeteria, or other school settings.

Support Physical Activity

Encourage your child to engage in regular physical activity at school and provide any necessary accommodations or modifications to ensure their safety and well-being. Communicate with physical education teachers, coaches, and extracurricular activity leaders about your child's diabetes management needs and any precautions or limitations they should be aware of.

Address Bullying and Stigma

Be proactive about addressing bullying and stigma related to diabetes at school. Educate classmates, teachers, and school staff about diabetes to promote understanding, empathy, and inclusivity. Encourage open communication and create a supportive environment where your child feels comfortable discussing their diabetes management needs and concerns.

Communicate Effectively

Maintain open and ongoing communication with school staff, including regular check-ins, updates, and discussions about your child's diabetes management plan, progress, and any changes in their health or medication regimen. Provide contact information for parents or guardians and healthcare providers, and encourage school staff to reach out with any questions or concerns.

Advocate for Accommodations

Advocate for reasonable accommodations and support services to meet your child's needs and ensure their safety and success at school. This may include access to a school nurse or health aide, permission to carry and self-administer diabetes supplies and medications, extra time for blood sugar checks or restroom breaks, and flexibility with scheduling or academic assignments during times of illness or medical appointments.

Promote Inclusion and Empowerment

Encourage your child to advocate for themselves and participate fully in school activities, clubs, sports, and social events. Foster a sense of independence, confidence, and resilience by empowering your child to manage their diabetes effectively and navigate challenges with courage and determination.

By working collaboratively with school staff, educating others about diabetes, and promoting self-care skills and empowerment, parents and caregivers can help children and adolescents with diabetes thrive at school and achieve their full potential. Remember to stay informed, involved, and proactive in advocating for your child's health and well-being in the school setting.

Parenting a child with diabetes comes with unique challenges and responsibilities, but with the right support and guidance, you can help your child thrive while managing their condition. Here are some ways you can support your diabetic child:

Educate Yourself

Take the time to learn as much as you can about diabetes, including its causes, symptoms, treatment options, and management strategies. Stay informed about the latest advances in diabetes care and research to better understand your child's condition and how to support them effectively.

Open Communication

Foster open and honest communication with your child about their diabetes. Encourage them to ask questions, express their feelings, and share any concerns or challenges they may be facing. Create a safe and supportive environment where your child feels comfortable discussing their diabetes management needs and seeking help when needed.

Empower Your Child

Empower your child to take an active role in managing their diabetes and making decisions about their health. Teach them age-appropriate self-care skills, such as checking blood sugar levels, administering insulin, counting carbohydrates, and recognizing symptoms of hypo- and hyperglycemia. Encourage independence and self-confidence while providing guidance and support as needed.

Provide Emotional Support

Living with diabetes can be emotionally challenging for children and adolescents, so it's important to provide emotional support and encouragement. Offer reassurance, praise their efforts, and celebrate their successes, no matter how small. Be a compassionate listener and validate their feelings, while also providing practical guidance and solutions to help them cope with any difficulties they may encounter.

Model Healthy Behaviors

Set a positive example for your child by modeling healthy behaviors and making nutritious food choices, staying physically active, managing stress effectively, and prioritizing self-care. Create a healthy and supportive home environment that promotes overall well-being for the entire family.

Work as a Team

Collaborate closely with your child's healthcare providers, including doctors, nurses, dietitians, and diabetes educators, to develop and implement a comprehensive diabetes management plan. Stay engaged in your child's medical care, attend appointments together, and advocate for your child's needs and preferences.

Establish Routine and Structure

Create a consistent routine and structure for managing diabetes at home, including regular meal and snack times, bedtime routines, medication schedules, and blood sugar monitoring routines. Consistency and predictability can help your child feel more secure and confident in managing their diabetes.

Provide Practical Support

Offer practical support to help your child manage their diabetes effectively, such as preparing nutritious meals and snacks, organizing diabetes supplies and medications, scheduling medical appointments, and assisting with blood sugar checks and insulin administration as needed.

Promote Independence

Encourage your child to develop independence and self-reliance in managing their diabetes as they grow older. Gradually delegate responsibility for diabetes tasks, such as checking blood sugar levels or adjusting insulin doses, and provide guidance and supervision as your child learns to manage their condition independently.

Stay Positive and Hopeful

Focus on the positives and celebrate your child's strengths, accomplishments, and resilience in managing their diabetes. Stay positive and hopeful about the future, and reassure your child that with proper care and support, they can live a happy, healthy, and fulfilling life despite having diabetes.

By offering love, support, and guidance, you can help your child navigate the challenges of living with diabetes and empower them to thrive while managing their condition. Remember that you are not alone in this journey, and there are resources, support networks, and healthcare professionals available to assist you every step of the way. Together, you and your child can face diabetes with courage, resilience, and optimism for a brighter tomorrow.

Chapter 14: Conclusion: Living Well with Diabetes

Embracing a Diabetic Lifestyle

Living with diabetes presents unique challenges, but it's also an opportunity to embrace a healthier and more mindful lifestyle. By making positive changes to your diet, physical activity, and overall approach to wellness, you can manage your diabetes effectively and enjoy a fulfilling life. Here are some key principles for embracing a diabetic lifestyle:

Focus on Whole, Nutrient-Dense Foods Emphasize whole, nutrient-dense foods in your diet, such as fruits, vegetables, whole grains, lean proteins, and healthy fats. These foods provide essential nutrients, fiber, and antioxidants that support overall health and help regulate blood sugar levels.

Balance Carbohydrates

Pay attention to carbohydrate intake and choose carbohydrates that are low on the glycemic index and high in fiber, such as whole grains, legumes, fruits, and vegetables. Aim to spread out carbohydrate consumption evenly throughout the day to prevent blood sugar spikes and crashes.

Practice Portion Control

Be mindful of portion sizes and practice portion control to avoid overeating and maintain stable blood sugar levels. Use measuring cups, food scales, or visual cues to help you portion out your meals and snacks appropriately.

Stay Hydrated

Drink plenty of water throughout the day to stay hydrated and support overall health. Limit sugary beverages and opt for water, herbal tea, or sparkling water instead. Staying hydrated can help regulate blood sugar levels and prevent dehydration, a common concern for people with diabetes.

Engage in Regular Physical Activity

Incorporate regular physical activity into your daily routine to improve insulin sensitivity, manage weight, and promote cardiovascular health. Aim for at least 150 minutes of moderate-intensity aerobic activity per week, along with muscle-strengthening activities on two or more days per week.

Monitor Blood Sugar Levels

Keep track of your blood sugar levels regularly and work with your healthcare provider to establish target ranges for fasting and postprandial (after-meal) blood sugar levels. Monitoring blood sugar levels allows you to identify patterns, make adjustments to your diet and lifestyle, and detect any fluctuations that may require medical attention.

Manage Stress

Practice stress-management techniques such as deep breathing, meditation, yoga, or tai chi to reduce stress and promote relaxation. Chronic stress can affect blood sugar levels and overall health, so it's essential to find healthy ways to cope with stress and prioritize self-care.

Get Plenty of Sleep

Prioritize good-quality sleep by maintaining a regular sleep schedule, creating a relaxing bedtime routine, and practicing good sleep hygiene. Aim for 7-9 hours of sleep per night to support overall health and well-being, as inadequate sleep can affect blood sugar control and increase the risk of complications.

Seek Support

Surround yourself with a supportive network of family, friends, healthcare providers, and fellow individuals living with diabetes. Connect with support groups, online communities, and resources to share experiences, gain knowledge, and find encouragement on your diabetes journey.

Stay Positive and Flexible

Approach diabetes management with a positive attitude and a willingness to adapt to changing circumstances. Recognize that managing diabetes is a journey, not a destination, and be open to learning, growing, and making adjustments along the way. Celebrate your successes, no matter how small, and be kind to yourself during challenging times.

By embracing a diabetic lifestyle that prioritizes healthy eating, regular physical activity, stress management, and self-care, you can live well with diabetes and enjoy a full and fulfilling life. Remember that every small step you take toward better health and well-being matters, and you have the power to make positive choices that support your diabetes management and overall wellness. Embrace the journey, stay resilient, and live each day to the fullest, knowing that you are capable of thriving despite diabetes.

Continuing Education and Advocacy

Living well with diabetes is an ongoing journey that requires dedication, resilience, and a commitment to lifelong learning and advocacy. As you navigate the challenges and opportunities of managing diabetes, it's essential to stay informed, engaged, and empowered to make informed decisions about your health and well-being. Here are some ways you can continue your education and advocate for yourself and others living with diabetes:

Stay Informed

Stay up-to-date on the latest research, guidelines, and advancements in diabetes care and management. Follow reputable sources of information, such as professional organizations, healthcare providers, and reputable websites, to access reliable information about diabetes prevention, treatment, and self-care strategies.

Attend Diabetes Education Programs

Participate in diabetes education programs, workshops, and support groups to learn from experts, connect with peers, and gain practical skills and insights for managing your diabetes effectively. These programs often cover topics such as nutrition, physical activity, medication management, blood sugar monitoring, and emotional well-being.

Engage with Healthcare Providers

Foster open and collaborative relationships with your healthcare providers, including doctors, nurses, dietitians, diabetes educators, and mental health professionals. Schedule regular check-ups, ask questions, and seek guidance and support to address any concerns or challenges you may be facing in managing your diabetes.

Advocate for Yourself

Advocate for your own health and well-being by speaking up about your needs, preferences, and goals related to diabetes management. Be proactive in seeking access to quality healthcare services, diabetes supplies and medications, insurance coverage, and support resources that can help you live well with diabetes.

Educate Others

Share your knowledge and experiences with diabetes with others to raise awareness, promote understanding, and combat misconceptions about the condition. Educate family members, friends, colleagues, and community members about diabetes prevention, management, and the importance of healthy lifestyle choices.

Participate in Research

Consider participating in clinical trials, research studies, or community-based initiatives aimed at advancing diabetes research, treatment, and prevention efforts. Your participation can contribute valuable data and insights that may help improve outcomes for people living with diabetes in the future.

Support Advocacy Efforts

Get involved in advocacy efforts to raise awareness, promote policy changes, and improve access to diabetes care and resources in your community and beyond. Join advocacy organizations, participate in advocacy campaigns, and lend your voice to initiatives that seek to address the needs and priorities of people living with diabetes.

Stay Positive and Resilient

Stay positive and resilient in the face of challenges and setbacks related to diabetes management. Focus on the progress you've made, celebrate your successes, and practice self-compassion and self-care to maintain your physical, emotional, and mental well-being.

By continuing your education, advocating for yourself and others, and staying engaged in the diabetes community, you can play an active role in improving outcomes and quality of life for people living with diabetes. Remember that you are not alone in this journey, and together, we can work towards a future where everyone affected by diabetes can live well and thrive.

Finding Support and Community

Living with diabetes can sometimes feel overwhelming, but you don't have to face it alone. Finding support and connecting with others who understand what you're going through can make a world of difference in managing your diabetes and living well. Here are some ways to find support and build a supportive community:

Join Support Groups

Consider joining a diabetes support group, either in-person or online. These groups provide a safe and welcoming space to share experiences, ask questions, and offer and receive support from others who are living with diabetes. You can find support groups through local community centers, hospitals, or online platforms dedicated to diabetes support.

Connect with Peers

Reach out to friends, family members, or colleagues who have diabetes or who have experience supporting someone with diabetes. Connecting with peers who understand the challenges and triumphs of living with diabetes can provide empathy, encouragement, and practical tips for managing your condition.

Participate in Online Communities

Explore online communities and forums dedicated to diabetes support and education. Websites, social media groups, and online forums can connect you with a diverse community of individuals living with diabetes worldwide. You can share your experiences, ask questions, and learn from others in a supportive and non-judgmental environment.

Attend Diabetes Events and Workshops

Look for local or national diabetes events, workshops, and conferences where you can learn from experts, connect with others, and discover new resources and strategies for managing your diabetes. These events often feature educational sessions, networking opportunities, and exhibits showcasing the latest diabetes products and services.

Seek Professional Support

Consider seeking support from healthcare providers, such as doctors, nurses, dietitians, diabetes educators, and mental health professionals. These professionals can offer personalized guidance, resources, and tools to help you manage your diabetes effectively and address any concerns or challenges you may be facing.

Involve Your Loved Ones

Involve your family members, friends, and loved ones in your diabetes journey. Educate them about diabetes, its management, and how they can support you in your efforts to live well with the condition. Open communication, empathy, and teamwork are essential for building a strong support network.

Volunteer or Give Back

Consider volunteering with diabetes advocacy organizations, nonprofits, or community groups that support individuals living with diabetes. Giving back to the diabetes community can be a meaningful way to connect with others, make a positive impact, and contribute to the greater good.

Practice Self-Care

Prioritize self-care and activities that nourish your mind, body, and spirit. Engage in activities that bring you joy, relaxation, and fulfillment, such as hobbies, exercise, meditation, or spending time in nature. Taking care of yourself is essential for maintaining your overall well-being and resilience in the face of diabetes.

By finding support and community, you can empower yourself to navigate the challenges of living with diabetes with confidence, resilience, and optimism. Remember that you are not alone, and there are many resources, connections, and opportunities available to help you thrive despite diabetes. Reach out, connect, and embrace the support of others as you continue on your journey to living well with diabetes.

Looking Ahead: The Future of Diabetes Management

As we look to the future, there is great promise and optimism for advancements in diabetes management that will continue to improve the lives of those affected by the condition. From innovative technologies to groundbreaking research, here are some key areas shaping the future of diabetes management:

Continuous Glucose Monitoring (CGM) Systems

Continuous glucose monitoring (CGM) systems have revolutionized diabetes management by providing real-time data on blood sugar levels throughout the day and night. Advances in CGM technology, such as improved accuracy, longer wear times, and integration with insulin pumps and other devices, are making it easier for individuals with diabetes to monitor and manage their blood sugar levels more effectively.

Closed-Loop Insulin Delivery Systems

Closed-loop insulin delivery systems, also known as artificial pancreas systems, are designed to automate insulin delivery based on real-time CGM data, reducing the need for manual insulin adjustments and minimizing the risk of hypo- and hyperglycemia. As these systems become more advanced and widely available, they have the potential to transform diabetes management and improve outcomes for people with type 1 diabetes.

Precision Medicine and Personalized Therapies

Precision medicine approaches are tailoring diabetes management strategies to individual patients based on their unique genetic makeup, metabolic characteristics, lifestyle factors, and treatment responses. By targeting treatments to specific subgroups of patients, precision medicine holds the promise of optimizing diabetes care and improving outcomes while minimizing side effects and complications.

Regenerative Medicine and Beta Cell Therapy

Regenerative medicine approaches are exploring the potential to restore insulin-producing beta cell function in individuals with type 1 diabetes through techniques such as beta cell transplantation, stem cell therapy, and gene editing. While still in the experimental stages, these therapies offer hope for a cure or long-term remission of type 1 diabetes in the future.

Lifestyle Interventions and Behavioral Support

Recognizing the critical role of lifestyle factors in diabetes management, there is growing emphasis on lifestyle interventions and behavioral support programs to promote healthy eating, physical activity, weight management, stress reduction, and other lifestyle behaviors. Integrating these interventions into diabetes care can help prevent or delay the onset of type 2 diabetes, improve glycemic control, and reduce the risk of complications.

Telemedicine and Digital Health Technologies

Telemedicine and digital health technologies are expanding access to diabetes care and support services, allowing individuals to connect with healthcare providers remotely, access educational resources and self-management tools online, and track their health data using mobile apps and wearable devices. These technologies offer convenience, flexibility, and personalized support for managing diabetes anytime, anywhere.

Advancements in Diabetes Education and Support

There is a growing recognition of the importance of diabetes education and support in empowering individuals to manage their condition effectively. Future advancements in diabetes education may include innovative approaches such as virtual reality simulations, gamification, peer mentoring, and culturally tailored programs to engage and empower diverse populations affected by diabetes.

Research and Collaboration

Continued investment in diabetes research, collaboration among multidisciplinary teams of scientists, healthcare providers, industry partners, and patient advocates, and partnerships with government agencies, nonprofit organizations, and philanthropic foundations are essential for driving progress in diabetes management and finding solutions to the complex challenges posed by the condition.

As we embark on this journey into the future of diabetes management, it's important to remain optimistic, proactive, and engaged in shaping the direction of diabetes care and research. By staying informed, advocating for innovation and progress, and supporting efforts to improve diabetes prevention, treatment, and support services, we can work together to create a future where everyone affected by diabetes can live well and thrive.

THANKS FOR READING

www.ingramcontent.com/pod-product-compliance
Lightning Source LLC
Chambersburg PA
CBHW051057250726
48656CB00001B/346